D1477849

Autism

A Holistic Approach

THIRD EDITION

DR MARGA HOGENBOOM
AND BOB WOODWARD

Floris Books

An important note:

The advice in this book may complement but should never replace speaking directly to a medical specialist. If you are concerned about your child's health, please consult a medical doctor.

The phrase 'Image of Man', used in reference to Steiner's holistic understanding of the human being, is intended to include both masculine and feminine genders, in the same sense as 'mankind'. Occasionally, where unavoidable and in historical quotes, the male gender has been used inclusively to acknowledge the fact that the ratio of boys and girls with autism is approximately three or four to one.

Historical texts and quotes may contain terms that are no longer used, but which were not considered inappropriate at the time.

Names of students in case studies have been changed for confidentiality.

In memory of Hans Müller-Wiedemann

First published in 2000 by Floris Books
This third edition published in 2013
© Dr Marga Hogenboom and Bob Woodward

Dr Marga Hogenboom and Bob Woodward have asserted
their right under the Copyright, Designs & Patents Act 1988
to be identified as the Authors of this work

All rights reserved. No part of this publication may
be reproduced without the prior permission of
Floris Books, 15 Harrison Gardens, Edinburgh
www.florisbooks.co.uk

 This book is also available
as an eBook

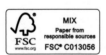

British Library CIP Data available
ISBN 978-178250-000-1
Printed in Great Britain
by TJ International Ltd, Cornwall

Contents

Contributors   9

Foreword   11

Preface   19

Acknowledgments   21

I. Background and Medical Research   23

    1. What is Autism?   25

    2. Possible Causes   37

II. An Anthroposophic Understanding of Autism   57

    3. Anthroposophy and Child Development   59

    4. Autism seen Anthroposophically   77

III. Interventions and Alleviation   97

    5. Some More Mainstream Interventions   99

    6. The Curative Educational Approach   109

    7. A Curative Educational Case Study: James   127
      Bob Woodward

    8. Autism and the Senses   157
      Mari Sterten

    9. Intensive Interaction Case Study: Anna   179
      Paula Jacobs

10. Art Club Case Study: Ralph, Mark and Oliver 189
    Réka Tóth

11. Ways Forward   197

IV. Source Material from Hans Müller-Wiedemann   207
    12. Early Diagnosis and Practical Advice
        for Parents   209
    13. The Topsy-Turvy World: An Anthroposophic
        Understanding of Autism in Early Childhood 227
    14. The Curative Educational School: Observations
        and Aims   243
    15. Curative Educational Therapy: Exercises in the
        Realm of the Four Body Senses   263

Appendix   273
    1. Additional Anthroposophic Background   275
    2. Further Therapies and Medical Treatments   285
    3. Useful Organisations   289

Bibliography   293

Index   309

Contributors

Dr Marga Hogenboom van den Eijnden, MRCGP (Utrecht)

Marga Hogenboom works as a General Practitioner at the Camphill Medical Practice near Aberdeen and specialises in anthroposophic medicine. She has lived and worked with children and adults with autism for the last thirty years, and was a member of the NICE Guideline group for autism in adults 2010–2011.

Bob Woodward, M.Ed., M.Phil.

Since 1970, Bob Woodward has lived with and taught children with severe learning difficulties, including children with autism, at The Sheiling School, Camphill community, in Thornbury, Gloucestershire.

Dr Hans Müller-Wiedemann, MD, Ph.D.

During the 1960s, Dr Karl König, the founder of the Camphill movement, asked Hans Müller-Wiedemann specifically to develop an anthroposophic understanding of children with autism, and to investigate how to help these children become socially integrated. Dr Müller-Wiedemann took up this task in earnest over some thirty years, and became an acknowledged and respected authority in this field. He published various books and articles about his work, as well as poetry. He died in 1997.

Johannes M. Surkamp, MBE

For many years Johannes Surkamp was the Principal of Ochil Tower, a Camphill Rudolf Steiner school for children with special needs in Perthshire, Scotland. He has worked in Camphill schools and villages since 1952, and was awarded the MBE in 1995 for his services to education.

Mari Sterten, BA Curative Educational

Mari Sterten is a therapeutic practitioner with 35 years experience of working as a teacher and therapeutically with children with special needs. She has a post-graduate diploma in Autism and a post-graduate certificate in Sensory Integration. She is a long-term co-worker at Camphill School Aberdeen.

Paula Jacobs, BA Social Pedagogy

Paula Jacobs has worked at Camphill School Aberdeen for six years. She has a BA in Social Pedagogy and a post-graduate certificate in Autism and Learning. She works as an assistant house co-ordinator and leads sessions of therapeutic play with children.

Réka Tóth, BA Social Pedagogy

Réka Tóth has lived at Camphil for seven years, supporting individuals with a variety of additional needs in educational, therapeutic and care settings. She has a BA in Social Pedagogy and a post-graduate certificate in Autism and Learning.

Foreword: Helping Autism with Knowledge of Human Nature

Infants and children with autism remind us how subtle the natural beginning state of mental life is, and how it depends on human sympathy. What is this consciousness, emotion and sympathy for human company which an infant can show?

After thirty years work as an infant psychobiologist I am sure that our fundamental motives require a profound revision of the scientific explanations accepted by mainstream psychology over the past century. I am, therefore, willing to listen to alternative accounts that claim to be comprehensive. I am especially interested if they also claim to have useful applications in the education of the young, or in therapeutic work with people of any age who are emotionally disturbed and have difficulties in thinking, learning and communicating with others.

What prevents experts from grasping essential motive principles in the naive? What kind of approach would be more successful? Must it be scientific, and if so in what way? Scientists have to concentrate on one line of enquiry, paying close attention to the often very delicate and difficult methods they use to get evidence. Their notions or *models* of reality deliberately reduce their view, in order to see their subject clearly and have some predictable influence over it.

Common sense can readily find shortcomings in the more contrived explanations, which often seem only able to see what a person can acquire by education or through the conventions of social institutions, art, literature, technology, logic and science. Sympathy and compassion, which are so important in the actual experience of family and life in a close community, in caring for the sick and in teaching, are intuitive and spontaneous. They are not easily explained in terms of external facts and information understood. The understanding mind in itself has moral impulses that have to be accepted without reasoned explanation.

Infants are inarticulate, unskilled and unsophisticated. They have no authority and no justifiable beliefs or opinions. However, as the research of the past few decades has brought to light, they do have purposes, interests and moral emotions. They perceive other people's actions and imitate. They perceive their mother's voice from before birth and attend to the musicality and narrative impulse of human talk and songs before they can see well. They engage purposefully with objects and events in the world around them and explore the effects of their body moving. They soon attend closely to interests and tasks that can be shared, seeking to grasp the meaning of the shared world. All this is achieved in the first year, much in the first few months, long before language and independent walking (Trevarthen 1987).

Many, perhaps most, academic authorities, including leading developmental psychologists, represent the infant as an impressionable learner, who, with little mental activity at first, has to acquire awareness of a self with a body and consciousness; who has to learn to perceive the independent life of other people with their bodies and consciousness. This psychology conceives the newborn as a scarcely conscious being whose emotions are crude states of agitation or arousal within the physiology of the brain and body, and are undifferentiated with regard to the reactions and identities of other people. More and more, this rational constructivist position, which sees the body as innate but the mind as learned, has had to revise its models. It has had to grant greater intuitive psychological powers to the infant, even from the moment of birth, and thus, inevitably, from before birth too.

True, the rapid growth of a child's consciousness and skill that takes place in the first years of life obviously occurs with amazing speed. From day to day babies become more aware and productive in response to their family and society, and then toddlers pick up the words that name the most interesting things and actions in the talk around them. However, this learner is from the start an active one, seeking companionship from people who accept his or her own vitality, curiosity and emotional enthusiasm. Learning to be clever in human society takes a human effort in the learner, and only a human child can contribute this active interest.

Children with autism have lost some of this natural vitality of mind, some of the intricate proficiency of acting and attending, of sensing the body and the world. As infancy passes there are higher hurdles to climb and a confusion of awareness, which toddlers with autism have to overcome in achieving confidence in their feelings of self, and finding the right methods of communication to make others understand and share (Hobson 1993). The main task is to attract sufficiently patient, supportive and receptive attention from those who give care and teach.

In this book, Marga Hogenboom and Bob Woodward have brought together a valuable fund of wisdom from members of the Camphill movement who have many years experience in therapeutic communities. In these residential settings they guide youngsters with autism to come to terms with their bodies and with a world that is more incomprehensible than it should be, and especially baffling in that essential human element on which meaningful learning depends.

The authors present a very readable account of the special features of children with autism, which I find to be accurate and comprehensive. Case reports clearly illustrate how the principles of anthroposophy are applied in practice. The lectures and articles by Dr Hans Müller-Wiedemann trace the development of a child through stages of mastery in engagement with an elusive reality and in communication. They also follow how a youngster with autism develops in spite of disjointed senses and incoherent or compulsive impulses to act, which themselves form a distorting barrier between the child and the world. Dr Marga Hogenboom brings her medical training to confront the problems children with autism have inside their bodies, and the possible effects of diet on their psychological life.

As with many who use a sympathetic intuition and direct experience to guide their therapeutic work, these authors are suspicious of, or sceptical about, brain-based explanations. Clearly they believe that reference to current brain science is reductive, and likely to miss psychological events that can be experienced and worked with. But all the links and dependencies that they so carefully record – between the digestive system and the mind; between bodily feelings and imagination or learning; between self-knowledge and sensitivity for other people's intentions, interests and feelings – are mediated by the brain, if we but knew how. And brain science is changing. At least some of those who are concerned with the richness of normal consciousness, or with the changes brought on by brain injury, neural disease or developmental disorder, are clear that some unifying principle operates and that emotions are integral to its operation (Damasio 1999).

Those of us who have filmed and analysed how infants come to the human condition with such eager anticipation and sensitivity are convinced that there is a coherent intentionality and intersubjectivity, or sense of 'self-with-other', from birth and before. The challenge is to understand how it gains in strength, discrimination, knowledge, skill and moral astuteness, while remaining whole and in sympathetic resonance with other human beings.

The authors of this book refer to evidence that youngsters with autism have been missing something from the start, and that this lack gradually becomes more obvious and worrying to parents and others, including peers, in the early years, especially the second and third years. As I have indicated, I do not believe we should take this account, with which I concur, as evidence that the human mind is incoherent at birth. Although subtle signs of detachment and turning inward can be discovered in retrospect in the life record of a child with autism, it remains unlikely that autism will ever be reliably diagnosed in early infancy. And that beginning of an active human spirit gives us hope.

Why take the emergence of a child's strength, skill and discrimination to be signs of construction of the mind from ground zero? Perhaps this idea reflects a weakness, a vanity in our whole culture's sense of the human condition, which is evident in psychological science and medicine. I believe it comes from too much faith and admiration for the training or instruction intended to make us accomplished citizens – skilled in movement, rational, articulate, literate and prosperous in a worldly sense. What is it to be humanly spiritual? Is it not to be biologically, essentially human – to be unsophisticated yet powerful in natural terms? I see all infants, including those developing autism, as being like this. In that, I believe, I am at one with the authors of this book.

Science does change our view of reality, and cognitive science and brain science are actively doing that now, but there is a price to pay for new expertise, dependent as it is on worlds that are technically strange, and remote from ordinary experience and common sense. The Western world changed after Darwin and Copernicus. Philosophers, too, also change our ways of living, and the post-classical philosophers of education in particular – including Comenius, Rousseau, Froebel and Steiner – upheld the human needs of children against projects of utilitarian instruction that may push them too hard or too early into a conventional mould.

With all the influences of our education, we remain both constrained and inspired by natural motives, and the motives of children are astonishingly strong. They are strong, too, when they are unusual, as in the case of children who become isolated and obsessional in their toddlerhood, and remain distant from the activities of their peers. They remain cut off in a world that becomes increasingly their own, unless others are sensitive to the need for companionship that they still possess, and that they greatly enjoy when the opportunity arises. This chance depends on sympathetic, playful and imitative approaches by people whose consciousness has gone through many stages of education, but who can still forgo levels of skill and sophistication to share the fundamental human impulses of what anthroposophy calls the 'spirit'.

Having recently reviewed treatments, therapies and educative regimes for children with autism, I would say this (Trevarthen, Aitken, Papoudi and Robarts 1998). Those methods that work best set out to meet the individual child's motivations and enthusiasms, such as they are, directly. They accept the expressions and actions of children with all their puzzling incoherence and fixations, emotional frailty and weak empathy, but also perceive their times of spontaneous ebullience, courage and affectionate appreciation of sympathetic care and fun. They realise that if there are to be beneficial changes in the child, changes have to come about in the responsiveness of parents, siblings, therapists and teachers – changes that will foster interest, enjoyment and learning. I see that accepting a 'holistic' or inclusive attitude to humanity in all children, as well as respect for their individualities, brings improvements. I contrast this with the academic identification of specific deficiencies at a higher, more educated level of mental functioning, which are all measurable by controlled pre-structured tests. While these tests, models and theories certainly illuminate puzzles that arise in the exploration of pathological effects that develop in the psychology of different groups of children, they have remarkably little practical use in helping these children. Every technique of intervention that does help has made direct engagement with the motives of the child for noticing things, feeling with people, and striving to have consistent effects in action, however weakened these motives may be. There is always a vitality that can be engaged. That is where one must begin.

Steiner's 'inner spiritual resources' are not *hidden* or *slumbering* in the infant. Nor are they lost in our purposeful rational selves. They remain efficiently active beneath the surface of all practicality, productive co-operation and explicit language. The moving body needs to be made to work as a whole, mechanically pacing and ordering the dynamic forces of mass and inertia of its parts harmoniously, co-operatively and economically, with little error or waste energy. The intelligence that understands what is perceived and that deploys special senses at the right moment and to the right place, is an agent of the impulse that moves the body, and that emotionally evaluates the risks and benefits of every intended action. All these are manifestations of the spirit of a person's living.

The coherence in time and space of these outputs of the mind – of the brain in its body – challenges the ambitions of human sciences, be they behavioural, psychological, cognitive, linguistic, physiological, biochemical or 'brain science'. Increasingly, all these different disciplines have, in a sense, had to become less disciplined, less confined within special paradigms and models, and more ready to take in evidence from the wide field of human natural history, the arts and common experience. Human minds have general emotional and emotive powers which are both spiritual and intelligent (Donaldson 1992).

This book has taught me that the philosophical approach of anthroposophy, aiming to be guided by a comprehensive 'knowledge of the nature of man' clearly does inspire carers and teachers. It helps them take human concern for the life difficulties of children who feel unsure in their bodies, are out of firm touch with earthly reality, disorganised in their senses, especially the sense of shared meaning, and unable to conceive of the sympathy and companionship extended by parents, peers and teachers. They find the human spirit in children, in the sense of a unified purpose and consciousness, and identify in what ways it is frustrated by unclear representations of how to intend and what to expect of the world.

I admire this approach and am impressed with what I hear about achievements in the Camphill therapeutic communities, where staff, parents and companions of teenagers with autism enter into communication at many levels besides the rational and pragmatic.

Colwyn Trevarthen
Professor (Emeritus) of Child Psychology and Psychobiology
The University of Edinburgh

Preface

Autism is one of the most intriguing conditions of our time. It is unsettling to meet children and adults with such outstanding problems of social interaction. It puzzles us because it challenges the essential core of every human being – how to relate to our fellows.

For the last seventy years, work has been continuing with children and adults with autism in residential settings based on curative education and social therapy. These places have developed their work according to the holistic knowledge of the human being, as originally described by Rudolf Steiner (1861–1925) in his science of anthroposophy.

Since the first edition of *Autism: A Holistic Approach* was published in 2000, the amount of research, theories and discoveries has avalanched; autism is the focus of many researchers. There are three directions in which the evolving understanding of autism is focused. The medical-scientific world is still mainly searching to understand autism as a brain disorder, which is genetically determined. Parents realise that their children are also having physical symptoms of distress and problems with their digestion, in the form of constipation, diarrhoea and food sensitivities. Many high functioning people with autism describe sensory and sensory integration problems.

These three aspects are slowly starting to form a coherent whole, and sensory problems are now clearly recognized in the DSM-5 (The American Psychiatric Association's *Diagnostic and Statistical Manual*, in its fifth edition). You can say that our book was ahead of its time in 2000, with its clear emphasis on sensory integration.

Chapters 1, 2 and 5 have been updated to reflect new methods of diagnosis and approaches in mainstream medicine, a new chapter on the sensory aspect of autism has been added (Chapter 8), and new case

19

studies from social pedagogical settings have been included (Chapters 9 and 10). The rest of the book remains largely unchanged.

We would like to dedicate *Autism: A Holistic Approach* to Dr Hans Müller-Wiedemann, who died in December 1997, and was an outstanding pioneer in the field of autism research, based on his comprehensive understanding of anthroposophy. His work was published mainly in German, and has remained mostly unknown to English readers.

Dr Müller-Wiedemann spent many years of his life living with children and young people with autism, in several therapeutic communities belonging to the worldwide Camphill movement. I met him for the last time in 1996 at a medical conference in Switzerland, where the sensory experience of children with autism was discussed. Dr Müller-Wiedemann was already frail and only able to attend part of the conference. However, he still managed to make an inspiring contribution regarding the lack of secure bodily experience in children with autism, and how to remedy this.

The authors hope that this book will stimulate the open-minded reader, whether a person with autism, a parent or a professional, to consider a new point of view. This book does not claim to provide all the answers, but hopes to contribute to the research, discussion and development in the field of autism.

Dr Marga Hogenboom

Acknowledgments

The authors would like to thank Johannes M. Surkamp MBE. for his translations from the original German of the four articles by the late Dr Hans Müller-Wiedemann (see Part IV). The authors are grateful to Verlag Freies Geistesleben, Stuttgart, Germany for permission to publish translated versions of three articles (Chapters 12, 13 and 14), previously published in *Der frühkindliche Autismus als Entwicklungsstörung* (1981). Chapter 15 originally appeared as 'Neue Aspekte der Förderung Autistischen Kinder' in *Autismus Heute Band 2*, Verlag Modernes Lernen, Dortmund (1990). Again the authors are grateful for permission to reproduce a translated version of the text.

Bob Woodward's contributions have largely been selected his 1997 M.Phil. thesis entitled *Autism in the Light of Anthroposophy*.

Thanks to the children described in the case studies, and to their parents for permission to refer to their developmental histories and work with them. Bob is also grateful to his colleagues at the Sheiling School, Camphill community who fully supported this research project.

Thanks also to Hazel Townsley for her professional skills on the word processor. This new edition could not have happened without the thoughtful editing of Sally Polson.

I.

BACKGROUND AND MEDICAL RESEARCH

1. What is Autism?

During the second half of the twentieth century, since Leo Kanner's (1943) first description of the syndrome he termed 'early infantile autism', many people have sought to explain the symptoms of autism. This search has given rise to important observations and investigations of children with autism, made at biological, psychological and behavioural levels (Happé 1994). This data has in turn generated a divergency of theoretical interpretations of causation, but as Baron-Cohen and Bolton (1993) point out, there is still no clear-cut answer as to the cause, or perhaps causes, of autism. This chapter will focus on the phenomenology which enables us to suspect or recognise that a child has autism, and will then examine the key criteria for gaining a formal diagnosis.

Phenomenology

Biographical accounts written by parents of children with autism provide telling first-hand descriptions of the typical features of the condition (Lovell 1978, Park 1983, Hocking 1990, Kaufman 1976), which appear during the first three years of life. They are evident in the marked indifference and aloofness of these children towards other people. The following examples, from these four biographies, illustrate this important and central autistic characteristic.

Simon was about nine months old, and apparently physically perfect, when his mother, who was pregnant with her second child, began to feel anxious about her first-born son. These anxieties arose through observing Simon's rate of development and that of a friend's little girl who was of the same age. In comparison Simon seemed much slower and too placid and '...seemed to take no interest in the world around him' (Lovell 1978, 4).

Moreover, he did not make eye contact with others. By the time he was 21 months old, Simon showed a marked indifference towards his peers and also towards his new baby sister. When he was three and a half years old Simon was seen by a paediatrician at the local hospital, and, after observation and tests, the mother was told that, 'Simon is autistic' (Lovell 1978, 18).

Elly, the fourth child of Clara Park, smiled at seven weeks, later made eye contact, and reached out for objects at the usual time. She sat at nine months and only learned to walk when about two years old. However, it was not late motor milestones which concerned her parents, but rather Elly's marked lack of response to their spoken requests during her second year. Physically nothing seemed to be amiss, but the beautiful two-year-old child took no notice of other people. Describing a seaside holiday, Park writes that Elly was:

> ...a bronzed, gold baby of unusual beauty walking
> along the sand. She might have walked straight ahead,
> deliberately swerving to avoid an occasional collision,
> without a backward look, forever, so little did she need of
> human contact. (Park 1983, 5)

Sam was the first child of a mother who, during and after pregnancy, was often anxious and stressful. He smiled at five weeks and physically seemed to be developing normally. However, Sam did not look at his mother, nor did he reach out for things later on. By ten months he could sit, but it was impossible to catch his attention person to person. Towards the end of his second year, Sam did not respond to anything his mother said, and appeared unable to understand language. He rarely looked at anyone, or only with an indirect glance. In the course of his third year, his parents sought medical advice from Dr Elizabeth Newson, an expert on autism. After observing Sam and interviewing his parents, she remarked that, '...he does present as a rather classically autistic child' (Hocking 1990, 37).

Raun, the third child of Barry and Suzi Kaufman, appeared to be perfectly healthy at birth, and was given an APGAR rating of ten.* However, during the first month at home he cried day and night and was unresponsive when held or fed. He developed a severe ear infection that needed antibiotics, which resulted in dehydration and urgent hospitalisation in intensive care. Fortunately, Raun recovered well and during his first year was a beautiful baby who smiled, laughed and played.

However, from one year of age Raun became more and more aloof, and by eighteen months eschewed human contact and communication: 'When Raun turned to you, he turned through you as if you were transparent'. (Kaufman 1976, 23)

An interview with medical and psychiatric professionals confirmed that Raun was showing 'autistic behaviour patterns'.

Typical characteristics

An overview of the four biographies quoted above reveals the following autistic features:

- Aloofness and indifference towards others, including parents and peers.
- Looks *through* other people.
- Avoids eye contact.
- Treats others like an object or tool.
- Lacks communicative intent via sound, speech or gesture.
- When speech is present appears to lack comprehension.
- Shows a marked preference for sameness and routine.
- Engages in repetitive and obsessional actions.
- Lacks interest to reach out and explore the surroundings.

* APGAR rating: a method of assessing the general state of a baby immediately after birth. A maximum of two points is given for each of the following – breathing, heart rate, colour, muscle tone and response to stimuli. A baby scoring ten points would be in optimum condition. When the score is low, the test is repeated at intervals as a guide to progress.

- ❋ Shows fascination for inanimate objects to be manipulated or put in order.
- ❋ Has no overt imaginative play.
- ❋ Shows little, if any, normal imitation.
- ❋ Displays unusual reactions to sensory stimuli.
- ❋ Is not deaf.
- ❋ Often musical.
- ❋ Good rote-memory.
- ❋ Able with jigsaw puzzles and has good visual-spatial skills.
- ❋ Physically good-looking, even beautiful, and often demonstrates co-ordinated and skilful movements.

All these typical features, as movingly described by the children's parents, are also confirmed in Wing 1996, Chapter 4. It is clear that children with autism appear either soon after birth, or at least by their third year of life, to be withdrawn and cut-off from their closest human surroundings. However, although their typical features are well known, historically the formal diagnosis of autism has not been entirely straightforward.

Diagnosing autism

The Kanner criteria

In the United States, Leo Kanner (1943) was the first person to describe autism when he identified eleven children as a distinct diagnostic group, who showed strikingly similar behavioural symptoms. Foremost among their symptoms was their '...inability to relate themselves in the ordinary way to people and situations from the beginning of life' (Kanner 1943, 242).

Kanner chose to label the cluster of behaviours that united these eleven children as 'early infantile autism', and concluded that:

> We must, then, assume that these children have come into the world with innate inability to form the usual,

biologically provided affective contact with people, just as other children come into the world with innate physical or intellectual handicaps. (Kanner 1943, 250)

Although Kanner's original paper (1943) lists ten diagnostic points, in a later, joint paper with his colleague, Eisenberg, they were reduced to the following five features:

1. Extreme detachment from human relationships.
2. Failure to use language for the purpose of communication.
3. Anxiously obsessive desire for the maintenance of sameness, resulting in a marked limitation in the variety of spontaneous activity.
4. Fascination for objects; handled with skill in fine motor movements.
5. Good cognitive potentialities.

(Furneaux and Roberts 1979, 41)

By 1955, when they had seen more than 120 such children, Kanner and Eisenberg isolated just two primary diagnostic features for autism:

1. Extreme self-isolation (or aloneness).
2. Obsessive insistence on the preservation of sameness.

However, since then, there has been considerable further debate.

Post-Kanner

In England in 1960, a committee chaired by Dr Mildred Creak was convened to examine diagnostic criteria. They listed nine points describing the condition of childhood schizophrenia, which at that time was a term that included 'childhood psychoses' and early infantile autism (Schreibman 1988, p.29). The first of the Creak points was:

'Aloneness and apparent lack of any social skills' (Furneaux and Roberts 1979, 24).

While this was considered essential to a diagnosis of autism, views differed about the key relevance of the other eight features. In any event it was rare that all nine features would be seen in children said to be autistic. Notably, and in contrast to Kanner, the Creak committee acknowledged impairments in the intellectual functioning of these children. However, individuals with autism differ in their degree of intellectual impairment as well as in the severity and combination of their other symptoms.

Schreibman points out the historical vicissitudes that have accompanied the diagnosis of autism:

> A major result of the evolutionary process of diagnosis,
> of the appearance of different sets of diagnostic criteria,
> and of differing motivations for diagnosis (e.g. research,
> education, economic considerations), is that diagnosis
> is not applied in a consistent manner. This has resulted
> in a tremendously heterogeneous population of autistic
> children. (Schreibman 1988, 33)

This very heterogeneity has led professionals to refer to a continuum, or *spectrum*, of autistic disorders (Wing 1993 & 1996), with Kanner's autism seen as a sub-group. Clearly, however, if the diagnostic goalposts are moved at different times and for different reasons, there will be more or fewer children identified, and as Wing points out, epidemiological studies of the prevalence of such children do in fact give widely differing figures: 'A few studies have strictly applied Kanner's criteria of severe lack of affective contact (social aloofness) and insistence on elaborate repetitive routines, and they found four to five children in every 10,000' (Wing 1996, 61).

The National Autistic Society estimates a prevalence of autism in the UK of one in a hundred. Gillian Baird (a paediatrician) and her colleagues surveyed a population of nine and ten year-olds in the South Thames region. They screened all the children who were known to have social and communication disorders, a special education statement or were diagnosed with autism. They used the ICD-10 criteria (see below and overleaf). The prevalence was 1.16 in a hundred children. (Baird *et al.* 2006) This is the same as the US, were one in 88 children has been diagnosed with autism. A recent research project in a town in South Korea, where all seven to twelve year-olds were screened, found an incidence of one in 38 (Insel 2012). It is clear that autism is very prevalent, and becoming a real international child health issue.

What then are the currently accepted core criteria for diagnosing autism?

Core symptoms of autism

Since 1978, two well-documented and internationally accepted medical diagnostic systems have been in use. These are:

1. The World Health Organisation's International Classification of Diseases, now in its tenth version (ICD-10).
2. The American Psychiatric Association's Diagnostic and Statistical Manual, in its fifth edition (DSM-5).

Since 1980, both of these systems have included the notion of the 'triad of impairments', regarded as common to individuals with autism spectrum disorder. For example, in ICD-10:

> Childhood autism (F84.0): Impaired or abnormal development must be present *before* three years of age, manifesting the *full* triad of impairments in:
> 1. Reciprocal social interaction.
> 2. Communication.
> 3. Restricted, stereotyped, repetitive behaviour.
> (Trevarthen *et al.* 1996, 11)

Today this term is considered to be negative and is not widely used, but the core symptoms for diagnosing autism remain the same. The

NICE (National Institute for Health and Core Excellence) Guidelines for autism in adults, 2010–2011, describe the core autism symptoms as:

* Persistent difficulties in social interaction.
* Persistent difficulties in social communication.
* Stereotypic (rigid and repetitive) behaviours, resistance to change or restricted interests.

However, in practice, definitive diagnosis requires considerable experience and expertise, for as Wing points out:

> Diagnostic problems arise because the triad can be shown in many different ways. Unless the diagnostician is fully aware of the triad of impairments underlying autistic conditions, s/he may be confused by a whole series of variables that affect the outward manifestations... (Wing 1993, 5)

Writing of the necessity for careful differential diagnosis when autism is associated with any other physical or psychological disabilities, Wing (1993) emphasises the importance of obtaining a detailed, early developmental history for each child. It is also important to have descriptions of the child's behaviour and responses in a variety of different settings, not just in the doctor's or psychologist's clinic. The NICE Guidelines for children with autism describe the diagnostic process in some detail. The assessment will start with detailed discussion of the presenting concerns and details of the child's experiences of home life, education and social care. The developmental history will focus very much on aspects of the ICD-10 or DSM-5, and there are autism specific tools for this. Observing the child is important and looking at possible different diagnoses. Medical and family history will be considered, as well as past and current health conditions. A physical examination is important, and further imaging or blood tests are only carried out when there is a specific question to assess.

Even though, according to Wing (1996), the precise age of onset of autistic behaviours may not be an essential criterion for diagnosis, the core autism symptoms are typically manifest by the second or third year. The tremendous developmental significance of the first three years of life will be highlighted later, when we interpret autism on the basis of anthroposophy. Meantime, it is noteworthy that for children with autism, 'It is significant that their insensitivity to other persons' feelings, purposes and experiences appears before the child is three years old, and after an early infancy that was apparently almost normal' (Trevarthen *et al.* 1996, 24).

DSM-5 and the end of Asperger syndrome

After several years of revision, the fifth edition of the American Psychiatric Association's Diagnostic and Statistical Manual of Mental Disorders (DSM-5) superseded the fourth edition (DSM-IV) in May 2013. Many conditions are described differently in the new edition and the changes in autism are quite specific. The DSM-IV described 'autistic spectrum disorders' (ASDs), including Autistic Disorder, Asperger's Disorder, and Pervasive Developmental Disorder Not Otherwise Specified (PDD-NOS). But from May 2013 onwards, the distinction between Asperger syndrome, autism and other conditions will no longer be used. There will be only one diagnosis, namely Autistic Spectrum Disorder (ASD).

Three different severity levels are described, levels 1, 2 and 3. They will depend on the level of support a person needs, due to their communication challenges and restricted behaviours and interest (Compart 2012).

The main reason for change is that there is not sufficient evidence for the distinction between Asperger syndrome and autism. Different doctors make different diagnoses and this affects the validity. Professor Francesca Happé states that Asperger syndrome may not be different from high functioning autism (Happé 2011; Whitehouse 2012). It is hoped that the change will lead to more consistent diagnosis.

Another significant change in the DSM-5 is the recognition and importance of sensory issues in autism. In the diagnostic framework, communication and social interaction will merge, while sensory experiences will be included alongside rigidity of thought (Muggleton and Seed 2011).

Here are the official criteria for diagnosing Autistic Spectrum Disorder, as approved by the American Psychiatric Board of Trustees on 1 December, 2012. The changes were made after considerable research and debate, and are based on expert opinion:

Must meet criteria A, B, C, and D:

A. Persistent deficits in social communication and social interaction across contexts, not accounted for by general developmental delays, and manifest by all three of the following:

1. Deficits in social-emotional reciprocity; ranging from abnormal social approach and failure of normal back and forth conversation through reduced sharing of interests, emotions, and affect and response to total lack of initiation of social interaction.

2. Deficits in nonverbal communicative behaviours used for social interaction; ranging from poorly integrated verbal and nonverbal communication, through abnormalities in eye contact and body language, or deficits in understanding and use of nonverbal communication, to total lack of facial expression or gestures.

3. Deficits in developing and maintaining relationships, appropriate to developmental level (beyond those with caregivers); ranging from difficulties adjusting behaviour to suit different social contexts through difficulties in sharing imaginative play and in making friends to an apparent absence of interest in people.

B. Restricted, repetitive patterns of behaviour, interests, or activities as manifested by at least two of the following:

1. Stereotyped or repetitive speech, motor movements, or use of objects (such as simple motor stereotypes, echolalia, repetitive use of objects, or idiosyncratic phrases).

2. Excessive adherence to routines, ritualised patterns of verbal or nonverbal behaviour, or excessive resistance to change; such as motoric rituals, insistence on same route or food, repetitive questioning or extreme distress at small changes.

3. Highly restricted, fixated interests that are abnormal in intensity or focus; such as strong attachment to or preoccupation with unusual objects, excessively circumscribed or perseverative interests.

4. Hyper- or hypo-reactivity to sensory input or unusual interest in sensory aspects of environment; such as apparent indifference to pain/heat/cold, adverse response to specific sounds or textures, excessive smelling or touching of objects, fascination with lights or spinning objects.

C. Symptoms must be present in early childhood (but may not become fully manifest until social demands exceed limited capacities).

D. Symptoms together limit and impair everyday functioning.

(Autism Resource Center of Central Massachusetts 2012)

These diagnostic changes are significant and will create some unrest, especially among people previously diagnosed with Asperger syndrome, who may not meet the new criteria. This could have implications for their funding and support services.

The central problem

As Kanner originally observed, it is precisely the inability of children with autism to relate socially with other people that remains the most pervasive and definitive feature of autism, and in a recent and thorough survey it was concluded that, 'The diagnostic or descriptive systems that we have reviewed affirm that autistic children have a primary inability to perceive others as people and to conceive what they may communicate' (Trevarthen *et al.* 1996, 24).

This conclusion, pointing as it does to a fundamental perceptual and conceptual inability and difficulty, is confirmed by the anthroposophic theory of autism presented in Chapters 3 and 4. This is particularly relevant in relation to the development and functioning of the child's higher senses of ego and thought, seen against a background of the incarnation processes of soul and spirit during the formative first three years. In Chapter 3 it will also become clear that disturbances in the typical steps leading to the experience of self-identity in young children, vis-à-vis their surroundings, should also be recognised as central to the autistic condition and the evident lack of social awareness and reciprocity.

Whereas children with autism's inability to make affective contact and relationships with others has long been acknowledged, the role of their own self-experience has not yet been fully appreciated.

In order to gain this appreciation it is not only necessary to view the question of 'What is autism?' on biological and psychological levels (Happé 1994), but also to include the spiritual level on which each child's essential being is to be found intact. In other words, we must aim for a holistic view that encompasses body, soul and spirit.

2. Possible Causes

Historical perspectives

According to Kanner (1943) autism is a condition, precipitated by the over-intellectual, emotionally inadequate and frigid characteristics of the child's parents. In 1956, Eisenberg and Kanner spoke of how, 'Emotional refrigeration has been the common lot of autistic children' (Bettelheim 1967, 389).

However, Kanner himself did not claim that 'refrigerator' parents were the sole cause of autism. Rather he believed that the pathology was present from birth, and was either a result of organic factors or, as Schreibman expressed it, of 'the interaction of organic predispositions with specific environmental events' (Schreibman 1988, 49).

Nevertheless, environmental and psychogenic factors were strongly advocated during the 1960s by the psychoanalyst, Bruno Bettelheim. He wrote that, 'Wherever infantile autism is viewed as an inborn impairment, of whatever variety, the resultant attitudes towards treatment will be defeatist' (Bettelheim 1967, 405).

These views express the polarisation which existed between advocates of the organic versus the psychogenic and the environmental schools of primary causation.

While Bettelheim did not accept the hypothesis that autism was due to an original organic defect, he did not however rule out the possibility of its later appearance: 'Actually, I believe that in earliest development, soma and psyche are so little differentiated that to a more enlightened time the entire controversy between organic and psychogenic hypotheses at that age may appear moot' (Bettelheim 1967, 403).

However, he still recommended the removal of children with autism from their parents, in order to provide them with a more supportive environment in which they could be helped to recover from their withdrawn and traumatised state (Baron-Cohen & Bolton 1993).

In the 21st century scientists are now striving to find a common cause, gene or pathway, which might explain autism. In his foreword to this book, Colwyn Trevarthen sums up the challenges scientists encounter when trying to understand consciousness and grasp the innate drive in human beings to communicate.

The understanding of autism is closely linked to these challenges. In general, autism is now firmly viewed as a neurodevelopmental disorder in the category of pervasive developmental disorders with a genetic basis. It is clear that autism is a complex disorder and that no single cause is likely to be found. This chapter gives a brief summary of the main areas of biologically orientated research, with a special emphasis on one of the latest hypotheses: that autism could be a metabolic disorder.

The reader has to be aware that everything described in this chapter is still in a state of flux, and according to modern evidence-based practice, autism is still *only* diagnosed by observation.

Genetics and autism

According to the newspapers genetics will soon be able to explain all human behaviour. The headlines speak about a gene for obesity and schizophrenia. This is, of course, an oversimplification. There is no direct relation between our genes and our behaviour, but it is clear that autism does have a genetic component. This has been found through twin and family studies. There are families in which two children have autism, or families where a parent has Asperger syndrome and a child has autism.

One of the indications that autism has a genetic component is from research with twins. Identical twins share the same genetic make-up, and there is a high risk of both twins having autism as opposed to nonidentical twins. The risk of both identical twins having autism varies from 36 per cent to 91 per cent. This was found in three epidemiological studies (Folstein and Rutter 1977 and 1988; Le Couteur, Bailey and Rutter 1989; Steffenbergetal 1989, in Harris 1995).

I knew two young ladies, identical twins both with autism, who had limited speech, hardly made eye contact and particularly enjoyed rocking backwards and forwards. However, they had completely different personalities: one was out-going and sanguine, and the other more serious and melancholic.

The genetic link is also visible in certain genetic syndromes, such as Rett's syndrome and tuberose sclerosis, in which there is a high incidence of autism. In these instances, the risk of having a second child with autism is higher than originally thought, and could be between three and five per cent, which is important for families to know (Connor and Ferguson-Smith 1997). In addition, the higher incidence of communication problems in non-autistic siblings of children with autism also points to a genetic component.

Autism Genome Project

Researchers into the genetic background of autism have started the Autism Genome Project (AGP). This is a large-scale, collaborative genetics research project that aims to identify autism susceptibility genes. Autism is a complex condition and its genetic architecture is not simple. This means that researchers will need many genetic samples of people with autism and strong scientific co-operation between clinical and laboratory researchers (Autism Speaks 2013a).

The researchers have published more than two hundred articles in scientific journals since 2003. One of those articles describes a genetic correlation in two subgroups of autism (Ledford 2010). The researchers looked at 1000 people with autism and compared them with 1300 people without autism, using imaging techniques. This new study demonstrated that subjects affected by autism tend to have more rare 'copy number variants' (CNVs) affecting their genes than the control individuals; the copy number variants are detected in less than one per cent of the population. Some of these mutations are inherited whilst others are considered as *de novo* or new because they appear in the patients but are absent in their parents. Researchers have noticed that in patients with autism, a large number of these mutations affect the genes already associated with autism or with intellectual disabilities.

Interestingly, Stephen Scherer from the Hospital for Sick Children in Toronto, one of the lead authors of the study published in *Nature*, is quoted as saying, 'We find that the genetic variations we discovered are actually rare in their frequency, meaning that most individuals with autism are actually probably genetically quite unique, each having their own genetic form of autism' (Connor 2010). This research tells us that genetic components could play a factor, but that they are not the same for different people with autism.

Robin P. Clark comments in his blog (June 14, 2010, www.autismcauses.info) that what the research found only accounts for a small percentage of autism cases. He still thinks that autism is a polygenetic condition just as IQ variance is polygenetic. So, in other words, there are so many genetic factors at play that it is not possible to identify an individual one. He thinks that researchers are starting at the wrong point and that genetics will never be able to provide the answer. He still thinks that research will show in the future that autism has a mainly environmental cause.

Autism and brain structure

Another area of great interest at the moment is the function of the brain. As autism can be seen as a brain dysfunction, are the brains of people with autism different from those of other people?

Research shows that the area of our brain that relates to emotions (the limbic system) is affected in some people with autism. This could have happened already during the embryonic period, but becomes visible around the age of two to three years.

Another part of the brain where abnormalities are often found in people with autism is the cerebellum, the smaller part of our brain relating to co-ordination of movement and the co-ordination of sense impressions (Courchesne 1991; Raymond, Bauman and Kemper 1989, in Harris 1995).

Post mortem research compared seven brain tissue samples from boys with autism to six brain tissue samples from boys of a similar age without autism. The children with autism were found to have on average 67 per cent more neurons (brain cells) than boys without autism. More specifically they found 79 per cent more neurons in the dorsolateral prefrontal cortex and 29 per cent more in the prefrontal cortex (Lainhart & Lange 2011).

This is interesting as the prefrontal cortex is associated with complex thoughts and behaviours, including language, social behaviour and decision making. The medial prefrontal cortex is considered to be important for social and emotional behaviour. The dorsolateral prefrontal cortex is important for planning, reasoning and more complex cognition.

Children without autism have around 1.16 billion neurons in the prefrontal cortex, children with autism 1.94 billion. This can explain why many children with autism have a relatively large head. Pruning of brain cells is an important part of development, normally happening between the ages of one and two, and this is possibly different in children with autism.

Autism and brain function

The emphasis is now veering towards research into brain function, which has been tested with modern imaging techniques. Some reports show that there is less co-ordination between the different regions of the brain in people with autism than in other people.

But what does this tell us? Although autism is regarded as a neurodevelopmental disorder, what is the cause of different neurological development? Brain development occurs primarily during the embryonic period and the first two years of life, and takes place through the multiplication and migration of nerve cells, although selective cell death is also important. However, this process of normal brain development can be disturbed.

From an anthroposophic point of view, the ego-organisation of a child is engaged in the development of the brain – or, in other words, our experiences and activities help to shape the brain. Therefore it is understandable that the natural development of the brain is affected if the ego is not properly integrated. In this book we work with the assumption that autism is an ego-integration problem. Thus the spiritual-soul being of the child can't sufficiently direct the bodily, sensory, emotional and intellectual development.

Some children clearly have previous or existing brain damage, and their lack of ego-integration can be caused by the difficulties of the ego in making use of the damaged instrument, as is the case in some secondary autisms.

Autism and neurochemistry

There are different chemicals, called neurotransmitters, such as serotonin, dopamine, adrenaline and endogenous opiates that affect brain function by passing neural impulses between different cells. Is autism caused by an abnormality in the function of one of the neurotransmitters?

Serotonin abnormalities have been found to play a role in autism, but there is no consistent abnormality found in all people with autism. Endogenous opiates (also known as endorphins) can play a role in all this, as they could influence all the neurotransmitters (Knivsberg 1997).

Autism and testosterone

Dr Baron-Cohen, one of the leading autism researchers in the UK, is assessing with his team whether levels of testosterone in amniotic fluid influence the likelihood of autism. They have found that the testosterone level of amniotic fluid is inversely related to social development, language development and empathy; and that foetal testosterone is positively associated with systemising and the number of autistic traits.

They are collaborating with the Statens Serum Institut in Copenhagen, Denmark to extend this study and test if elevated levels of foetal testosterone are associated with a later diagnosis of autism spectrum conditions.

The rationale for testing foetal testosterone comes from animal studies, which suggest that, prenatally, this hormone 'masculinises' the brain. Given the sex ratio in autism and Asperger syndrome (which are predominantly male conditions), and the masculinised cognitive profile reported in studies of empathy and systemising in people with these diagnoses, foetal testosterone may be an important biological mechanism to help understand the phenotype (Autism Research Centre).

Assessment of children with autism

The parent or carer reading all this would imagine that, by now, investigations into brain function or neuroimaging or metabolic investigations would be part of the assessment process. Despite the findings described above, neither genetic testing, nor EEG (measurement of electric activity of the brain), nor MRI scans support the diagnosis of autism. The NICE Guidelines for autism in children advise not to routinely perform any medical investigations as part of an autism diagnostic assessment, but only to do use them if there are clear indications. They recommend genetic testing if the child has dysmorphic (unusual) features or to perform an EEG when there is suspicion of epilepsy (NICE Guidelines for autism in children, 2011).

Autism and metabolism

Metabolism relates to the intake and digestion of our food. We are mostly unaware of these processes, but we become aware of them through experiencing discomfort, cramps, reflux or constipation.

Our digestive process starts the moment we smell or see food. We produce saliva, our gastric juices are stimulated and we feel hungry.

During chewing, the breakdown of carbohydrates starts in the mouth itself (Smith 1995). On swallowing, the digestion of proteins and fats commences in the stomach. After a couple of hours food is passed on to the small intestine, two important organs secrete digestive juices into the duodenum – the first part of the small intestine. The liver, on the right side of our body below the diaphragm, produces bile, which is a waste product of blood metabolism but also helps with the digestion of fats. The pancreas is situated behind the stomach and produces digestive juices, which help with the breakdown of protein and carbohydrate. The small intestine itself also produces enzymes that are involved in the digestion of sugars and protein.

Dr Natasha Campbell-McBride describes in detail how a healthy gut functions. She discusses the importance of this large, not often discussed organ in the gut: the intestinal flora, with most adults having between 1.5 and 2 kilograms of bacteria in their gut. This is an enormous amount. And they function in a highly organised way. This flora maintains the health of the gut wall and supports normal digestion, immunity and health. Fibre in our diet helps to maintain the balance of beneficial flora. Once this is out of balance and abnormal flora is present, fibre in the diet stimulates the abnormal flora, causing more discomfort. The abnormal flora also limits absorption of iron, causing different degrees of anaemia. Giving iron supplements in those cases only stimulates the growth of iron. When food is properly broken down it is absorbed through the wall of the intestines into the bloodstream.

How could the digestive process relate to autism?

Many parents noted that their children had not digested their food properly, and often had smelly bowel movements. Some children suffered from chronic constipation or diarrhoea. The parents mentioned it to their doctor, a stool sample was taken but a diagnosis was never made.

Other parents realised that their children reacted strongly to different foods. Parents experimented with diets and noticed that their children calmed down when milk, bread or other foods were excluded.

All these observations indicated that something in the digestive process might be disturbed. Those experiences stimulated research into the effect of diets and the digestive process in people with autism. In 1966, Dohan indicated a possible connection between food and mental health, and published his results in an article entitled 'Cereals and Schizophrenia: Data and Hypothesis'. A Norwegian scientist, Reichelt and his co-workers found an increased level of peptides (the breakdown product of protein) in urine collected over 24 hours from people with autism and schizophrenia. These peptides were in part breakdown products derived from gluten (found in wheat, barley, rye and oats) and casein (milk products).

Paul Shattock, a biochemist and the father of a child with autism, did extensive research in this area together with Paul Whiteley and others (Whiteley *et al.* 1999). They focused their research on digestive problems and developed a method to examine the morning urine of people with autism. An increased concentration of certain peptides was found. What did this mean? Based on these observations a hypothesis was developed – *autism as a metabolic disorder.*

Dr Campbell-Mcbride extends this concept. She describes two main problems.

Abnormal gut flora causes overgrowth of yeast and candida. Yeast requires glucose to function. Normally glucose gets transformed into lactic acid, water and energy through glycolysis. In people with yeast overgrowth, according to Dr Campbell McBride, this is different, and glucose is changed by the yeast into alcohol and acetyldehyde. In pregnancy this problem can worsen and this could affect the unborn child. She also points then to the opiate effect, as described below.

Despite exciting research theories, there is no overall explanation for brain abnormalities or the neurochemistry findings, and there is no explanation for the fact that some children seem to develop normally until eighteen months to two years of age, when suddenly their development stops and they even regress. I see many children who have followed this pattern.

It appears that something is primarily wrong with the digestive process in the gut. Food substances, especially proteins, are not properly broken down. Consequently, peptides permeate the gut, enter the bloodstream and even pass the blood/brain barrier (this is a fine barrier of blood vessels that protects our brain by trying to keep toxic substances out). These peptides manage to enter the brain where they then act as a neurotransmitter and have the same effect as endorphins (or opiates). Endorphins, which are substances with opiate-like effects, are produced by our body and, in our brain, help to create a feeling of well-being. However, if the level of opiate activity is raised due to other opiate-like substances then they make us high, restless or spaced out, with a poor ability to concentrate. They can also alter our sensory perceptions; we would see colours differently and our perception of our body would alter. Many of these symptoms can be found in people with autism. They are hyperactive, have a high pain threshold, and we now know from many personal descriptions, that their sensory impressions are fragmented.

Excess peptides in the blood are excreted by the kidneys and can be found in urine. Research has confirmed that people with autism can have different peptides in their urine compared with other people (Whiteley *et al.* 1999). Why are these peptides absorbed in a higher concentration by people with autism? This can be due to many reasons. In the gut there is a fine balance among the different enzymes, acidity and bacteria, which together maintain the health of the gut.

These peptides derive especially from milk products (casein) as well as from wheat, barley, rye and oats (gluten), and are seemingly not properly digested or broken down in certain people with autism. It is interesting that gluten is broken down to gluteomorphine and casein to casein morphine, which are peptides with opiate-like effects. The intestinal balance can be disturbed for different reasons:

1. There are not enough peptidase enzymes (which break down proteins), the acidity in the stomach is too low or there is a lack of vitamins and minerals.
2. The gut wall itself is too permeable through inflammation, caused by excess antibiotic use or candida infections.
3. The blood/brain barrier could be less effective because of a viral or bacterial infection or trauma.

The following children showed some of the problems discussed above.

EXAMPLE 1

Jamie was the second child, and seemed to develop normally until the age of eighteen months. He used some words, had good social interaction with his family, but then suddenly within a week he withdrew into autistic behaviour. He suffered frequently from ear infections that required treatment with antibiotics. When he arrived at our school at the age of six he was in total control of his bodily functions, and would pass water twice a day, but only opened his bowels when he was at home with his parents and wearing a nappy.

EXAMPLE 2

Brian was the second child in his family. His brother has Asperger syndrome. His development appeared normal until he was about fourteen months old. Overnight, he changed into a restless, aggressive boy who lost all his speech. He now has severe sleeping problems.

Whatever the reason for the metabolic disturbance in children, if the hypothesis is correct, there will be an elevated level of opiate activity in the brain, which will affect the perceptions, mood, behaviour and emotions of that person. The elevated opiate level in the brain could also affect brain development in a young child. During embryonic development and the first two years, there are many connections formed between different nerve cells in the brain. If this process is prevented or altered, brain dysfunction will arise.

I have discussed the effect of metabolic problems on the well-being and behaviour of children with autism through the effect of endorphins, but as a parent, carer and doctor it is vitally important to be aware of the possible pain and discomfort that gastro-intestinal problems can cause. For example, constipation can be quite distressing for a child and cause discomfort, sleeping problems and aggression.

A researcher investigated 36 children with autism who had gastro-intestinal problems (chronic diarrhoea, flatulence and abdominal discomfort and distension) by means of gastro-intestinal gastroscopy. It was found that 25 children had reflux, whereby food from the stomach enters and irritates the gullet; fifteen had chronic gastritis (an irritation of the stomach lining); and fifteen children had chronic duodenitis (Howard *et al.* 1999). This illustrates the point that we must be aware of medical problems in the gastro-intestinal tract of children with autism.

Therapies

Different approaches to remedy the metabolic, intestinal problem have been developed. Donna Williams, a woman with autism who has written extensively about her experiences, believes she is able to function properly thanks to a very restricted diet (Williams 1996).

Therefore, exclusion diets are one approach, and often mean the exclusion of gluten and casein. In the past few decades this approach has been studied scientifically on a small scale with convincing results. One study compared parents' observations of twenty children with urinary peptide abnormalities. Ten children followed a special diet and ten children did not. After one year, there was a significant reduction of autistic behaviour in the children on the diet, and no change of autistic behaviour in the control group. The different research projects are summarised in the article, 'A survey in dietary intervention in autism' (Knivsberg, Reichelt & Nodland 1999).

It is best to start a diet before a child is ten years old, as increased awareness of the diet can create tension. Also a diet should not be started light-heartedly, as it can be necessary for some children to continue with this diet for their whole lives. Some children react very negatively to the reintroduction of gluten or casein in their diet.

In Britain Paul Shattock and Paul Whiteley from the University of Sunderland have developed a protocol – known as The Sunderland Protocol – to give some guidance with exclusion diets (Shattock and Whiteley 2000). Their advice is to first remove casein from the diet for a three-week trial. In young children any change is usually visible in a few days, whereas in adults changes are seen after ten to fourteen days. The withdrawal effects are mostly short-lived, but can be severe in young children.

After three weeks gluten removal can be tried, which means the removal of wheat, barley, oats and rye from the diet. Gluten seems to need longer to leave the body so the effects are not so dramatic, and it takes up to four weeks to see any difference. Shattock and Whiteley suggest trying the diet for three months and then re-evaluating the situation. The withdrawal effects with gluten are milder but can last longer.

It is possible that other foods or additives could be the problem. Whiteley and Shattock recommend keeping a food diary to see if any particular food leads to a change in mood, sleeping or performance. To prevent nutritional deficiencies the support of a dietician during this process is also a good idea.

The protocol also discusses whether a particular yeast in the gut could be a problem because it may make the gut more permeable to certain foods. Shattock and Whiteley mention that some parents remove yeast from the diet, or treat the child with nystatin, an anti-yeast drug (this has to be prescribed by a GP).

All in all the area of food exclusion and possible supplements is not an easy issue and asks for a huge commitment and close observation of the child from parents.

It may be that the person is oversensitive to some food substances.

However, the reaction to gluten and casein is not an oversensitivity but a toxic reaction. This can be difficult to prove but an exclusion diet seems the most useful to determine this. A problem with exclusion diets is that people can become sensitive to foods that are used to replace the gluten or casein. If this happens, then after initial progress, a regression in behaviour is seen.

This seemed to be the case with Martin, a tense, restless but gentle 25 year-old man with autism. At certain moments he would become very aggressive and difficult, but really improved after the introduction of a gluten and dairy-free diet. He was calmer, more concentrated and had fewer outbursts. This suddenly changed after one year, and he became quite unsettled and aggressive. His diet had not changed, so it was suggested that he had become oversensitive to corn, which was used to replace the gluten in his bread.

Another problem is that any exclusion diet can be very antisocial and can result in a preoccupation with food and the person's diet. This was also a problem for Martin; he started to resent his diet and this created a lot of tension.

It is, of course, much simpler with young children who are not so aware of the food they receive on their plate. In some families everybody sticks to the diet to make it easier for the person with autism.

Understanding and Implementing Special Diets by Lisa Lewis is a practical book, which helps people to start this complicated diet and also provides recipes. Another more recently published title, *Diet Intervention and Autism* by Marilyn le Breton, offers another straightforward guide to this kind of diet (Lewis 1998; Le Breton 2001). There are other possible approaches with diets. Low sugar and low carbohydrate diets combined with anti-fungal treatment are used to treat the problems of candida (a fungal infection) in the gut, which is caused by repeated antibiotic use. Supplements with minerals and vitamins are another approach; the most commonly used are vitamin B6 and magnesium. Developments are very rapid in this field, and it is best to acquire the most current knowledge.

Dr Campbell Mcbride has a different approach to diet. Her advice is to give children with those problems mainly fish, meat, eggs, nonstarchy fresh vegetables, nuts and seeds, bean and pulses, honey and high quality fats – no grains or carbohydrates.

The real problem is to know which children or adults can benefit from a diet or supplements. The guidelines for possible diets are clear as described above, but there are no clear guidelines for other interventions as yet.

Possible indications for a metabolic approach could be:

1. Problems with digestion, such as constipation or diarrhoea, or a diagnosis of a bowel illness.
2. Regression into autism after normal development.
3. An increase in the urinary excretion of certain peptides, related to gluten or casein.
4. Strong family history of sensitivity to gluten.
5. Negative reaction to certain foods.
6. History of severe colic as a baby.
7. Black rings around the eyes.

I am connected as a GP to a school for children with special needs. Many children are on a diet, mainly started by the parents. It is clear that this is very helpful for some children.

WHAT DO MODERN SCIENCE AND DOCTORS THINK?

Modern science looks objectively at facts. Ideally something has to be shown in a large trial, where neither the patient nor the researcher knows which intervention is used. Dietary intervention has not been shown to be scientifically beneficial.

I was quite amazed at this, after all the stories from parents, books and articles. I asked the chairperson of the NICE Guidelines group, Dr Gillian Baird, what her experiences where. She said that diet was not proven to be helpful, but she knew children for whom it was beneficial.

Anthroposophic understanding

How, therefore, does this all relate to insights derived from anthroposophy? Ego-integration is a real problem for autism (see Part II for a full explanation of this term). It is clear that failed ego-integration will be noticeable on all levels of the human being: on the level of sensory integration; in difficulties developing empathy; and in problems with communication, social interaction and imagination.

One of the consequences of unsuccessful ego-integration is that digestion does not function properly. It is the task of the ego to break down food substances, which is done with the help of digestive enzymes.

Rudolf Steiner describes this process in a book he wrote with Dr Ita Wegman entitled *The Fundamentals of Therapy*. In Chapter 9, 'The Role of Protein in the Human Body and Proteinuria', he describes how protein is a living substance, made up of oxygen, nitrogen, hydrogen and carbon, and is full of life-giving forces.

When we eat we absorb protein. The digestive process starts in the stomach and is aided by pancreatic juice. Protein is an alien substance for our body, because it contains etheric life forces of another living being, namely, from a plant or an animal. The protein is broken down into peptides and amino acids, absorbed and used by the body to form our own protein. During this process, the life forces from the other organism are removed and the protein is integrated in the etheric forces of our own body.

Therefore, the protein has to be transformed in the digestive tract so that there are no alien etheric forces left. The protein has to become inorganic and lifeless so we can make it our own. The ego-organisation does this with the help of the pancreatic juice. A person needs an ego-organisation that is strong enough to digest protein and to re-integrate it in our etheric body. If not, then the protein will contain too much foreign ether from a foreign organism. The consequence is that the protein is excreted. This is a way of describing an allergy or intoxication caused by protein.

According to Steiner, healing results from the strengthening of the activity of the ego-organisation in the pancreatic juice. Steiner wrote this in 1924, and it is therefore fascinating in the light of recent research, which clearly shows that people with autism excrete certain peptides.

Steiner clearly put a lot of emphasis on the proper digestion of proteins. In 1924 he also gave lectures to co-workers who started to work with special needs children (Steiner 1998). Here, he discusses the importance of the relationship of chemical substances in protein and the profound effect they can have on the behaviour of children. He describes what happens if the metabolic limb system of a child is too weakly developed, and the albumen substance of the human organism is prevented from containing the right amount of sulphur. The consequence, according to Steiner, is that the child will have fixed ideas, starting from early childhood.

Recent research by Waring points to the possible importance of sulphurisation in autism (Waring 2000). The indications are that children with autism are deficient in the enzyme *phenol sulphur transferase*. This enzyme has two functions. Firstly, it ensures that mucous membranes are coated with mucous to protect them. Secondly, it helps to hydrolate toxins from the body – that is, surround toxins with extra water molecules. If a person does not have enough of this enzyme, toxins build up and the gut can become permeable to undigested proteins. In this instance, parents can add bath salts containing magnesium sulphate to their child's bath, which has had seemingly good results. It is interesting to note that in 1924, Steiner highlighted a link between sulphur deficiency and obsessive behaviour.

Anthroposophic treatment

The challenge for anthroposophy is to translate these insights into an anthroposophic medical treatment. The whole idea of exclusion diets is to remove foods that could cause problems for children. However, ideally we would like to strengthen children's digestive systems, so they can cope better and digest different foods.

In curative education the input from anthroposophically trained doctors has always played a central role in the education and treatment of children. Doctors working in the same field have used remedies to help children with autism with sensory integration, the development of emotional life (König 1953), or to help their ego become more incarnated (Klimm 1981).

The treatment of different metabolic organs has always played an important role in the treatment of children with autism. Potentised remedies have been used to stimulate the ego-organisation to incarnate in the metabolic system. Another approach has been to give compresses or specific massages to different organs. The aim of these treatments is to strengthen the working of the ego-organisation in its digestive activity. This can be done through strengthening liver function, stimulating pancreatic activity, and harmonising the activity of the gut.

Children have responded positively to the treatment. There is often a rapid response with regard to bowel movement, and a consistent, subsequent improvement in social interaction according to personal statements from colleagues. The following example illustrates the response:

Craig is a four-year-old boy with autism. He has severe diarrhoea, which is smelly and acidic. This was investigated but no diagnosis was made. He was started on a treatment of anthroposophic medication, and received Digestodoron tablets, which harmonise bowel function. He also received other remedies directed at activating the pancreas. He responded well, and his bowel movement improved. His behaviour also changed: he became less hyperactive; his eye contact improved; and after three months of treatment, he could speak in sentences (he already had some words) and said, 'Mummy, look at the clouds.' This shows a wish to share observations, an activity that is so often lacking in children with autism.

Development in this area is happening very quickly. I expect that our approach to autism and understanding of autism will progress in the coming years, especially with regard to the role of the metabolism in autism.

Conclusion

I have tried to show that the concept of autism as a metabolic disorder does not contradict the concept of autism as failed ego-integration. There are indications that, in certain children, autism could be caused by a disruption of the normal levels of endorphins. Insufficiently broken-down proteins can cause this disruption by having a disturbing effect on the development and activity of the brain.

If the ego is not fully integrated, it has profound effects on the developing child at all levels, and also on the working of the organs in the digestive tract. If the organs involved in metabolism do not work properly, food cannot be properly digested.

Anthroposophic medicine can support the activity of the metabolic organs with appropriate remedies, and so enable the ego to connect better with the metabolic system. It is important to know that this is just one aspect of the anthroposophic medical approach to autism and that more research is needed to evaluate this intervention.

Parents and therapists are working with different hypotheses regarding autism. The scientific world is still focusing on research into genes and brain function. The schism between brain, genes and gut is quite outspoken. My conclusion is that there is not one single cause for autism, even on a genetic level. There are probably many different causes. During the year 2010–11, I was part of the NICE Guidelines group for autism in adults. This is the leading scientific body in England and Wales, which collates all available medical research on a topic and, together with experts, makes guidelines for other professionals. It is disappointing to see how little evidence there is for any intervention or conventional medication. In my opinion, the future will bring the different areas of research together, as human beings are not only made of genes, brains or guts, but these are all integrated aspects of a whole person.

An anthroposophic interpretation of autism offers another explanation for the core autistic symptoms. This view recognises the intact spiritual being of each child, which is hidden behind any other psychological or organic factors (See Part II). It is important that investigations into possible causative factors for autism should be conducted on different levels (organic, psychological *and* spiritual), which co-exist and interact in the total human being. The reality of the child's essential spiritual nature should not be denied due to a one-sided focus on physical organic problems. Rudolf Steiner (1990b) often pointed out that an incomplete knowledge, in which the spiritual element was omitted, would inevitably lead to an erroneous view of material-physical processes.

II.

AN ANTHROPOSOPHIC
UNDERSTANDING
OF AUTISM

3. Anthroposophy and Child Development

Rudolf Steiner and anthroposophy

Rudolf Steiner (1861–1925) explained anthroposophy's Image of Man in his 35 books (Seddon 1988) and some six thousand lectures. At the outset it is important to stress that Steiner did not formulate theories, or even hypotheses. Instead, he claimed that what he described in his books and lectures was the content of rigorous scientific research, which had employed spiritual faculties of perception. Such spiritual faculties could, according to Steiner, be developed by anyone who was willing to undergo strict and systematic inner soul training and self-education (see Appendix 1).

> In every human being there slumber faculties by means
> of which he can acquire for himself a knowledge of higher
> worlds ... It can only be a matter of how to set to work to
> develop such faculties. (Steiner 1993, 19)

Steiner did not expect or want his readers or listeners to simply accept unthinkingly what he had discovered through his own methodical spiritual research. He did, however, expect a certain open-mindedness and freedom from prejudice from those who considered his work. He maintained that the results of spiritual-scientific research were accessible to lively thinking, and could be verified in the experiences of life itself.

The usual scientific way of obtaining proof or validation, via the independent replication of research findings and the power of predictions, was well known to Steiner, and he encouraged his pupils to undertake their own research on the basis of his indications.

It is clear that Steiner's spiritual-scientific findings are immensely practical and innovative from their applicability in many diverse fields (Davy 1975). Of these, education provides a striking example. Since the founding of the first Steiner-Waldorf school in Stuttgart, Germany, in 1919, Steiner-Waldorf education has become a worldwide movement with over one thousand schools and two thousand kindergartens in more than sixty countries.

Steiner's Image of Man

What then are some of the broad essentials of anthroposophy's holistic Image of Man, which underpins Steiner's concepts for new approaches in education, curative education, medicine, and also for an understanding of autism?

1. The human being is threefold in nature and consists of Body, Soul and Spirit. Each one of these principles is also clearly differentiated by Steiner in a threefold manner (Steiner 1973, Chapter 1). As Lievegoed (1993) explains, Steiner's tripartite Image of Man clearly contrasts all other models that have been influential in the twentieth century. This is mainly because other models have failed to recognise the essential spiritual being of man in its relationship to the psyche and the body. Needless to say, a purely biochemical or computer-like model of the human being completely rejects any independent reality for both the spiritual and soul principles. However, the soul, which functions in the three psychic forces of thinking, feeling and willing, is the mediator during earthly life between body (matter) and spirit. The human soul therefore receives influences from both the material world and the spiritual world as shown in Figure 1. The soul is the stage whereupon our manifold experiences are enacted.

One of the most far-reaching of Steiner's discoveries was the precise relationship and connection between the three psychic or soul forces

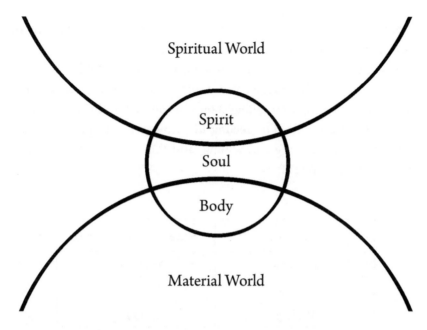

Figure 1. The soul as mediator between body and spirit.

of thinking, feeling and willing, and the bodily organism. After more than thirty years of spiritual-scientific research, he found that each soul force corresponds to a particular organic system (Harwood in Davy 1975). See Table 1.

Soul Force	Organic System
Thinking	The nerve-sense system, with the brain sensory organs. Principally centred in the head.
Feeling	The rhythmical system, with the organs of heart and lungs. Principally centred in the chest.
Willing	The metabolic-limb system, with all the organs below the diaphragm. Principally centred in the lower body.

Table 1. Relationship of the soul forces to the bodily organism.

61

Steiner was also aware that in the human body the functions of these three organic systems interconnect with each other.

Moreover, the three soul forces are active on three different levels of consciousness (Zeylmans van Emmichoven 1982), so that the conscious awakeness of thinking stands in contrast to the unconscious sleep state of the will. The feeling life, however, occupies a middle realm, between thinking and willing, and the consciousness there is dream-like. See Table 2.

Soul Force	State of Consciousness
Thinking	Awakeness
Feeling	Dreaming
Willing	Sleeping

Table 2. Relationship of the soul forces to different states of consciousness.

2. Each human being is, in reality, a spiritual being. This being is often referred to by Steiner as the 'ego', and it is important that this term is not confused with its usage in any totally different images of man (see Lievegoed 1993, Chapter 6 for a comparative survey of such images). For each of us, our true being or ego existed before birth, and will continue to exist after death. However, our ordinary day-to-day self-awareness, or ego-consciousness, is narrow and restricted in comparison to the transcendent nature of our true, or higher, ego.

3. Our being is partially subject to periodic re-embodiments, or reincarnation (Steiner 1973). The conscious impulse for this arises strongly during life in the spiritual world between our last death and the new, pre-planned, birth (Wachsmuth 1937; Steiner 1975). It is only by entering into earthly life once again that we can further evolve and mature.

4. However, when effecting a new incarnation on earth, human beings do not arrive as a tabula rasa. Instead they bring with them certain consequences from the actions and circumstances of their previous earth-lives, together with definite goals for the current life. Collectively this constitutes their personal karma. Karma, seen anthroposophically, is not however fatalistic, but can be realised in more than one way, and therefore allows for individual initiatives and for freedom: '...life can only be understood in its details if we can find how the various karmic influences are interwoven' (Steiner 1969c, 30).

5. The human being is engaged in a continuum of purposeful spiritual evolution and development, which involves complex processes of metamorphosis and transformation. Chapter 4 in Steiner (1989) describes in great detail the successive evolutionary stages of Man and World. When seen in this broad context, our modern, individualised and personal self-consciousness and reasoning ability are relatively recent acquisitions, and can lead us towards ever greater independence, freedom and a strong sense of moral responsibility.

6. The unique Christ Event (the life, death and resurrection of Christ), and the healing redemptive impulse that flows from it, was seen by Steiner as absolutely pivotal to the whole course of world evolution. He claimed that:

> All that was conferred upon human evolution through the coming of Christ, has been working in it like a seed ... We are but at the beginning of Christian evolution. (Steiner 1989, 218)

Steiner (1976b) perceived this Christian evolution as being inwardly linked to the development of individual ego-consciousness within human beings in modern times, and it therefore transcends any particular religious dogmas or beliefs.

It is important to emphasise, for our later understanding of autism, that the unique biography of each person develops karmically in relationship with others, and that the core of each individual is a spiritual being in the becoming (i.e. involved in a continuous process of evolution and further development), thoroughly imbued with meaning and purpose. Indeed, as individuals become more spiritually aware and awake, their sense of purposefulness increases because they can more clearly perceive their own standing in the stream of human evolution *per se*. On the basis of this broad anthroposophic background, we will now turn to child development.

Child development

According to anthroposophy, children as beings in the becoming have consciously set their own goals and aims for this particular life, long before they are physically born on earth (see Appendix 1). Child development is a differentiated process whereby the child's spiritual being, or ego, strives to incarnate into earthly existence in order to fulfil its personal karma in social relationships with others. We can call this process ego-integration. As Meadows observes:

> If it were possible for a child to grow up without any social
> relationships at all, and it probably is not, that child would
> not be recognisably 'human' – would not have spoken
> language, would not have the intellectual skills we revere,
> would not, probably, have self-awareness or empathy. Social
> interaction is necessary for all this... (Meadows 1986, 173)

Therefore it is clear that the process of ego-integration must take place within, and is indeed dependent on the children's social context with others. Fortunately, children are not normally conscious of the enormity of the leap they must make when crossing over from the spiritual to the physical modes of existence. As neonates, infants and young children literally sleep and dream their way into the surroundings of their new lives, which include their inherited bodies. The following quotation from Steiner vividly captures the importance, for children's well-being, of sleeping into their new, earthly situation.

When awake   When asleep

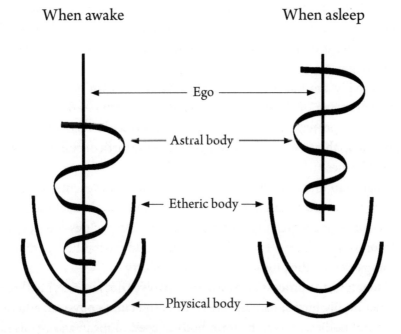

Figure 2. Man's fourfold constitution.

> ...if the child were still living in this pre-earthly
> consciousness his (new) life would be a terrible tragedy,
> a really terrible tragedy ... He had prepared himself
> according to his karma, according to the result of previous
> lives. He was fully contained within his own spiritual
> garment, as it were. Now he has to descend to earth
> [where] ... he clothes himself in a body that has been
> prepared by a number of generations. (Steiner 1982, 25)

This physical-material, hereditary body, then serves as a model
(Steiner 1972) on which the child's ego endeavours to form and
fashion its very own individualised body, according to karmic laws.
This organic building process takes approximately seven years to
complete, and is achieved through the use of certain formative
life forces, which Steiner often called etheric forces. In three
succeeding phases (see Steiner 1986, 111), these etheric forces

65

are gradually withdrawn, or freed, from their exclusively biological functions, and then become available on a different level, as soul faculties within the child; for example, as memory and mental image capacities.

Normally, around the seventh year, the child's own body has been built, and some of the etheric forces are metamorphosed into living, imaginative powers of thought, which are in no sense abstract. Steiner summed up this new step in development as the birth of children's own etheric bodies.

At around fourteen years of age, other new soul capacities emerge, leading to the formation of independent judgments, abstract thoughts and a much more personal feeling life. These capacities are due, in anthroposophic terms, to the birth of the child's astral body, and are accompanied by the physical changes of puberty.

Therefore, the process of incarnation involves not just one, but three distinct bodily births: namely, the birth of the child's physical, etheric and astral bodies. (Here, the term body is used to mean an organised and contained system of forces, not only a material-physical organism.) The full impact of these different bodily births and metamorphoses needs to be clearly understood by educators who are active in Steiner-Waldorf education (Steiner 1975a; Harwood 1982; Aeppli 1986; Lievegoed 1987; Childs 1991) and also by anthroposophic doctors (Bott 1982; Glöckler & Goebel 1990).

It is precisely through incarnation into these three bodies that the child's ego enters into earthly existence. Therefore, anthroposophy often refers to the fourfold constitution: namely, the ego with three bodies. It is important for us to note the following:

1. The physical-material body provides earthly building blocks (minerals also have physical-material bodies).
2. The etheric (or life) body not only underpins growth and reproduction, but is the bearer of memory and imagination in man. Organically, it functions through the glandular system (plants also have etheric bodies).
3. The astral (or soul) body enables sensations, inner

consciousness and ensouled movements to come about (that is, movements that are expressions of the soul through the physical organism, rather than mechanical movements). Organically, it functions through the nervous system (animals also have astral bodies).

4. The ego (or spirit), as the essential being of man, alone enables the process of individualisation of the three bodies in each person through ego-integration, self-consciousness and individual biography (Hansmann 1992). Organically, the ego functions through the warm blood system. (Only human beings have egos in earth existence).

In our attempts to understand autism in a new way, we realise that the ego of children with autism is unable to sufficiently penetrate into and individualise its three bodies. This shows itself a) in connection with the etheric body, in the children's lack of imagination; b) in connection with the astral body, in repetitive and compulsive movement patterns; and c) in respect of the ego itself, children with autism invariably fail to establish a secure and reliable self-consciousness.

With reference to human fourfoldness, Steiner (1990b) often pointed out that when we are awake the ego and astral bodies are united with the physical and etheric bodies. However, when we sleep, the ego and astral bodies are withdrawn from them and enter into a spiritual existence. We can illustrate these two situations, in a simple schematic way. See Figure 2.

Normally, when we wake up in the morning, the process of ego-integration takes place and we regain our self-consciousness, personal identity and conscious memory. However, when the ego and astral bodies are withdrawn during sleep, we lose our self-consciousness, personal identity and autobiographical memory. We shall see later that children with autism do not wake up properly to self-consciousness, nor do they easily go to sleep. This can be explained as a disturbed ego-integration in relationship to the three bodies.

Environmental factors

Steiner placed great emphasis on the social, moral and physical environment that surrounds and influences children throughout their early years. He said that we should think of the very young child as a single, highly sensitive and perceptive sense-organ (Steiner 1988). Everything children perceive in their surroundings, even the thoughts and feelings of people with whom they establish a close rapport, has a profound effect upon the reorganisation and active development of their own physical body from the inherited model body.

The marked sensitivity and acute vulnerability of young children to their environment derives from the faculty of imitation, to which Steiner gave considerable importance. In his educational lectures, he described the child before the arrival of teeth as, 'pre-eminently an imitative being' (see Appendix 1).

However, it is known that children with autism show marked difficulties in imitation compared to normally developing children (Hobson 1993, 72). As Wing states, 'Imitation is one of the skills that is basic to developing social behaviour, so its impairment is a significant part of the autistic picture' (Wing 1996, 50).

The first three years of life

While the acclaimed Swiss child psychologist, Jean Piaget (1982), was particularly concerned with the evolution of cognition in young children, a growing interest in the emotional and social development of infants has been seen in more recent years (Harris 1991; Dunn 1988). The sequential developmental behaviour of young children from birth has been observed and mapped since the 1960s (Sheridan 1988).

However, the nature of young children's inner experiences, and the quality of their varied perceptions, still remains a field for continued exploration and discovery (see Appendix 1). According to Karmiloff-Smith:

Lower senses ⟶ Higher senses	
Balance	Hearing
Word	Movement
Life	Thought
Touch	Ego

Table 3. Correspondences between the lower and higher senses.

> For a long time it was thought that the newborn perceives
> and interprets objects in a kind of chaotic, surreal way,
> famously described by the early twentieth-century
> psychologist, William James, as the infant's 'buzzing,
> blooming confusion'. But recent research suggests that the
> infant's world, although blurred, isn't that different from
> the adult's. (Karmiloff-Smith 1994, 47)

However, in contrast to this recent research, the inner process of
early child development can be seen, as Weihs (1984) suggests, as
effecting a withdrawal from an initially global and vague perceptual
field, towards increasing discrimination and objectifying of the world.
In other words, a contraction from a wide peripheric awareness
towards a centred and sharper consciousness, in which self and world
are increasingly separated. We shall see later that children with autism
retain something of this sensitive early peripheric consciousness,
instead of achieving a clear self-awareness and developing interpersonal
relationships with others.

In order to understand autism better we should take particular
note of the lower and the higher senses as characterised below (see
Appendix 1 for fuller explanation).

The four lower senses

König (1971) provides us with a detailed study of the lower senses from which the following brief accounts have been drawn.

Touch	gives us a first dim awareness of the boundaries of our bodily existence, and results in a sense of inner security and trust. Moreover, it is through touch that we can have a sense for the divine in the world; if a person had no sense of touch they would have no feeling of God.
Life	gives us a feeling of bodily well-being (or otherwise). Moreover, the initial feeling of self comes through the sense of life, with the experience of wholeness in our corporeality.
Movement	gives us an awareness of the co-ordinated movements and relative positions of our own body parts, and therefore of our integrated bodily existence.
Balance	gives us orientation in the three dimensions of space, and provides us with an enduring inner certainty.

It is specifically through the combined perceptions of the four lower senses that we can arrive at a sense of certainty of our own body and a complete body image. Together, these body senses give an existential and largely unconscious self-experience, which is distinct from an awake, sharp self-consciousness. However, if any one of the four lower senses does not function adequately, the very basis of our earthly existence can become uncertain and insecure, and we shall see later how this situation applies to children with autism.

The four higher senses

Steiner (1990b) gives very clear descriptions of these distinct cognitive senses.

Hearing   makes us aware of sounds and tones. It also
conveys the musical element of spoken language.
As such it already appears to function in the
embryo (Verny & Kelly 1982).

Word   makes us aware that a language is being spoken.
This awareness, according to Steiner, is distinct
from what is conveyed through hearing alone.

Thought   makes us aware of the thoughts of another person,
which may be conveyed to us via spoken or
written language, or gestures. The perception of
thoughts or concepts, and therefore also of sense
and meaning, is in reality a sensory, not a cognitive
thinking process.

Ego   makes us aware of the ego-nature of another
person. Through this sense, which is the most
spiritual of the twelve senses, another's essential
humanity is recognised. Steiner (1990b) precisely
described the functioning of this highest sense
within our interpersonal relationships.

It is through the co-ordinated functioning of the four higher senses that we are able to become truly social beings (König, 1990), who can communicate and learn to empathise with others.

Additionally, it is important to note that there are specific developmental relationships and correspondences between the four lower and the four higher senses, which are shown in Table 3 (p. 69, see Aeppli 1993). In brief, a healthy development of the higher senses depends on the proper functioning and maturation of the lower senses. This dependency is very important when we come to interpret childhood autism, precisely because such children appear to have some higher sense impairments or dysfunctions, resulting in a profound lack of social sense and awareness. This, therefore, also has implications for their lower senses.

Self-consciousness

It is commonly known that when small children learn to speak, they do not use pronouns in reference to themselves. They still refer to themselves by name: Johnny or Jane wants this or that. However, as Sheridan (1988) observes, by the age of two and a half years children are typically able to use the pronouns 'I', 'me' and 'you' correctly. By three years, they use both personal pronouns and plurals correctly and also most prepositions. They also ask many questions beginning 'what', 'where' and 'who'. How then does the child come to the realisation that, in language function, he is not only Johnny Brown, but also I? Is this knowledge arrived at by some intellectual inference or deduction, as is often assumed to be the case (Flavell 1985, 259)? Is there a totally different explanation for this phenomenon? Steiner asserted that the emergence of this pronoun was an outer expression of inwardly experienced self-consciousness: 'In the course of his development as a child, there comes the moment in the life of a man in which, for the first time, he feels himself to be an independent being distinct from the whole of the rest of the world' (Steiner 1973, 35).

Steiner (1973) emphasised a simple fact, which, in its uniqueness, is mostly overlooked. Namely, that while all of us can apply every other name that exists to its corresponding object, 'I' can only be applied and used by an individual speaking of his or herself. Therefore, when children in their third year begin to use 'I' properly and consistently, they begin to experience the continuity of personal, autobiographical memory, which forms the thread of their entire earthly life (see also Appendix 1).

It may also be possible that a child who, for some reason, does not speak, still arrives at consciousness of self. However, it seems that children with autism who can speak do not refer to themselves as 'I' in a normal and consistent manner, and, developmentally, this observation is very significant (Hobson 1993, 95–101).

Social context

Two important events stand out in the early evolution of reciprocal contact and communication, especially between mother (or other main caregiver) and baby. Firstly, the establishment of eye contact at around two to three weeks, and secondly, the baby's first smile at four to six weeks. König attaches great significance to this latter event.

> The soul of the child breaks through and greets the world
> with acceptance and joy. The child acknowledges its
> decision to become a citizen of the earth. (König 1994, 67)

However, we know from literature that the absence of eye contact and social smiling can be early indicators of the presence or onset of autism (see Appendix 1 for further explanation of the anthroposphical social context).

Play

The developmental importance of the stages of play for children's active integration into the world are now well recognised (Garvey 1991). It would not be going too far to say that play is one of the most important activities in a child's life. König once pointed out that children's spiritual being, the ego, leads them into earthly life through play.

Fantasy and imagination, pretend and social play, play with adults, siblings and peers: all of these constitute a creative and increasingly socially-shared world of transformations and metamorphoses. What could better accompany the parallel, inner transformation of the body during the first seven years? For children, play is as natural and vital as eating and sleeping. In the deepest sense, play during the first seven years is 'the preparation for life', and for later realising personal karma (Britz-Crecelius 1979). As Steiner remarked, 'The way in which such a young child plays is a clear indication of its potential gifts and faculties in later life' (Steiner 1986, 118).

Unfortunately, the lack of creative play and fantasy is a characteristic feature of infantile autism.

In conclusion

From the preceding sections on early child development, and according to anthroposophy's holistic Image of Man, we can now state that:

- ❋ Children undergo a process of incarnation, from a pre-birth spiritual existence to a post-natal earthly life.
- ❋ Children's spiritual being is active, via etheric forces, in the complete organic reconstruction of their own individualised body from the inherited model body. The brain is worked upon and refined in the first two and a half years.
- ❋ Children are, above all, extremely sensitive sensory and imitative beings; the more so the younger they are.
- ❋ In the course of the first year, children's lower or body senses develop, accompanied by existential feelings of trust and security. These are linked to the subsequent functioning of their higher or social senses.
- ❋ In the course of the third year, children first achieve individual self-consciousness and thereafter start to refer to themselves as 'I'. This is the result of an existential recognition of their own uniqueness, and is a crucial moment in their biography.
- ❋ There then follows the age of defiance, of self-assertiveness, and the continuity of autobiographical memory.
- ❋ Child development is integrated into, and dependent on, the social context. Early awareness is peripheric and at one with the soul surroundings.
- ❋ Creative play is an expression of the ego's incarnation process, and is instrumental for the later realisation of karmic intentions.

Two key concepts

Finally, underpinning all that has been discussed above, are two fundamental anthroposophic concepts. The first of these is expressed by the term ego-integration, which is defined by Hansmann as, 'The process of the spiritual individual entering through conception and birth into his body and the environment of family and nature, of folk and historic time' (Hansmann 1992, 165).

It is precisely through ego-integration that developmental processes of metamorphosis and individualisation are able to take place effectively in the growing child.

The second key concept centres on the very *raison d'être* for ego-integration. Only through incarnation into earthly existence can individuals achieve new steps in their own spiritual evolution (Steiner 1959). This means that man is still a *being in the becoming* (see Appendix 1).

If we keep these two far-reaching concepts in our minds, together with the understanding of child development presented in this chapter, we are now ready to propose an anthroposophic interpretation of early infantile autism.

4. Autism seen Anthroposophically

Typical three year olds display a vivacious interest in life. They have long since mastered standing on their own two feet and walking where they want in their active exploration and conquest of the new world. They can speak well and clearly communicate their basic needs, wishes and questions. They refer to themselves as 'I', and can be extremely self-assertive in word and action, determined to have their own way. They still sometimes imitate what they have seen their father or mother or other adults doing, irrespective of whether they approve of it or not. Their whole nature dictates that they follow the examples they have observed. At play, they are master magicians, whose power of fantasy can create and transform anything in their surroundings, whether they are alone or with other children. They show obvious affection and trust with familiar others, including younger siblings, and are generally emotionally responsive and alert to their social surroundings. Three-year-old children are, therefore, thoroughly active little people, expressing their full participation in a world they share with others, in their own increasingly individual ways. However, it is a strong inner drive for successful incarnation, for ego-integration into this new earth life that fuels all this visible outer involvement and expression. There are indeed important and pressing things that can only be done, learnt and achieved in this particular down-to-earth existence.

Hypothesis

What would happen if the invisible, yet normally empowering, drive for ego-integration were to break down and fail early in life? What would this mean for the hidden and complex processes of transformation and metamorphosis that underpin typical child development? What would this mean if outwardly the child appeared to be physically perfect, even beautiful in appearance, and was apparently organically undamaged?

Anthroposophically, assuming what we have already described of early childhood to be true, we could predict certain serious developmental consequences. However, in doing so we must be quite clear that these specific consequences are not due to any of the many afflictions or dysfunctions that can also disrupt the course of normal development, such as early encephalitis. We must be sure that they have their root on the deeper soul-spiritual level of the basic existential drive, the will impulse to enter into physical incarnation. Usually this drive is strong enough to withstand and surmount any early illnesses, accidents or traumas experienced by the incarnating soul-spirit of the child in the first years of life or later, without autism occurring.

Implications of an unsuccessful early ego-integration

1. The inherited model body is not sufficiently taken hold of and transformed by the ego, resulting in the poor development of one or more of the lower senses. This leads to an underlying lack of bodily self-experience, inner security and trust, and an incomplete body image. Thus the very ground of existence is missing.
2. The lack of development of one or more of the lower senses would lead to impairment or even non-functioning of certain higher social senses, resulting in an autistic inability to make sense of the world, especially other people.
3. The general sensory organ and the power of imitation, which are essential in developing the new individualised body and in early communication with the social environment, are either weakened or break down altogether. This inevitably results in isolation and aloneness.

4. The release and particularly the metamorphosis of etheric forces, which normally lead to the development of fantasy and imagination, and are expressed in the child's natural urge to play, are impeded. Therefore, these most child-like attributes are markedly absent in children with autism.

5. The motor achievements of talking and thinking, which are intimately linked with the senses of word, thought and ego, are seriously disturbed, or perhaps altogether fail to take place. This results in further isolation from and incomprehension of the human environment.

6. During the third year, the contraction of the initially wide peripheric consciousness of the infant towards a more centred self-consciousness does not fully take place. If spoken language has been attained, the use of personal pronouns, especially 'I', will either be missing or confused. This results in an inability to separate self from surroundings, and to establish a personal identity.

7. The failure to effect typical ego-integration shows in disturbed or deficient sensory functioning, as well as in an inability to establish secure self-consciousness through the continuity of personal, autobiographical memory. The most singular and dramatic effect of this is an almost total inability to integrate actively into the stream of social life and to establish reciprocal human relationships. Children appear alienated from their closest human surroundings and have, or will soon develop, autism.

By considering the complex evolution of the anthroposophic interpretation of autism, we can see how these implications of disturbed ego-integration are supported in theory. We shall include the work of König (1960), Weihs (1984), and Müller-Wiedemann (1988); all were informed by decades of direct practical experience and observations through living and working with children with autism in Camphill schools.

The evolving interpretation of autism

Dr Karl König

In 1960, Dr König gave two lectures on the theme of 'The Autistic Child'. After a review and consideration of the typical symptoms of autism, he came to the following initial conclusions:

- The inability of a child to integrate into the sense, the meaning, of the environment and social surroundings is not primarily due to a dysfunction of walking, speaking and thinking but to a dysfunction in the development of the three higher senses of word, thought and ego.
- The general organ of sensitivity whereby children especially perceive the people in their surroundings is, for one or another reason, not functioning.
- The ability to imitate is absent in these children.

In seeking the deeper reasons for these dysfunctions, König came to further important, yet still initial, conclusions:

The active power of imitation depends on the child's general sensory organ. (This seems reasonable, since children must first perceive something before they can imitate it.)

Imitation and the sensory organ are both intimately concerned with the as-yet unborn etheric body of the child. This etheric body only comes to full birth around the seventh year, and meantime is normally protected by what Steiner (1975) described as the mother's etheric envelope (or sheath or shell). König's view gains clear support when Aeppli points out that:

> Steiner often speaks of how the small child, approximately
> up to the fourth year, still possesses a kind of 'general
> organ of perception' in his etheric body ... The child

still possesses the liveliness of perception caused by the enlivening etheric forces in the sense processes. (Aeppli 1993, 46–48)

If before or soon after physical birth, this maternal etheric sheath is ruptured, this will directly affect the child's own unborn etheric body, and consequently the general sensory organ and power of imitation. König thought that such a rupture could be caused by a traumatic event, and an examination of the case histories of children with autism led him to conclude that, '...you never find an autistic child where you cannot elucidate very clearly a shock, an accident, an illness – something which disturbs this time of becoming and birth' (König 1960).

The overall effect for unborn children or infants would mean that they wake up prematurely in their consciousness, when they ought to remain healthily unconscious and asleep. The profound, formative power of imitation is only possible because children, in their expanded consciousness, sleep into their surroundings (see Steiner 1990b, 150). Therefore, it follows that if this sleeping into life is prematurely disturbed, so is the capacity for imitation.

Furthermore, König pointed out:

If you study what is thought today about child autism you will find one school which sees the whole thing purely organically – for the one the brain is damaged, for the other (school) certain psychological things are the cause and reason for the disturbance.

But where does psychology start in a baby without being at once organic. Where in a baby does an organic lesion start without at once having mental consequences. It is all one. 'If such a child wakes up too early, at once the whole body suffers' (König 1960).

Here, we are immediately reminded of Bettelheim's views on the intimacy of soma and psyche in earliest development (see Chapter 2).

Finally, and most importantly, Dr König saw autism as the reaction of the soul or being of the child towards difficult existential circumstances. König therefore considered the acknowledgment of the child's spiritual being to be absolutely essential for any real understanding of autism and its symptomatology.

Dr Thomas Weihs

In 1970, Weihs put forward a developmentally based interpretation of autism. He was not concerned primarily with the identification of possible underlying aetiologies which, he believed, could be heterogeneous – organic, psychogenic or environmental – and which needed to be diagnosed for each child individually. Rather his aim was to understand autism in the light of the first three years of normal child development, as illuminated by anthroposophy.

Weih's observations strongly emphasised the unique inner awakening to self-consciousness, from an earlier peripheric awareness. In essence, he proposed that the phenomenon of autism could be understood as a reaction of young children to the incipient, and potentially overpowering and threatening, emergence of their own self-hood.

> To sum up, the attempt has been made to interpret childhood autism as a panic-reaction to the moment when the ego first makes itself known to a child between his second and third years ... In consequence of the panic-reaction, there can develop avoidance of the realisation of the self. (Weihs 1984, 91)

In reference to children with autism who speak, Weihs stressed the significance of the well-known phenomenon of pronominal reversal (see also Wing 1996, 39):

> This transposition of the personal pronouns is perhaps the most unique and classical demonstration of the panic-reaction against the dawn of one's ego-experience. The failure to lodge the ego-experience at centre is probably the core of childhood autism. (Weihs 1984, 91)

Interestingly, Weihs remarked that among hundreds of histories of children with autism, he had only found a small number showing signs of autism in very early infancy. Whether or not early signs are observable (Muller-Weidemann, 1988, believed that this was frequently the case), recent literature certainly agrees that the characteristic symptoms of autism are typically seen by the third year. As we saw in Chapter 1, the ICD-10 definition of childhood autism clearly specifies the full manifestation of the core autism symptoms before three years of age. This is, therefore, in keeping with Weihs' particular interpretation of the unique significance of the child's third year.

Additionally, Weihs considered that first-born or only children were more likely to be at risk of showing an autistic reaction, because of their position of special responsibility in the family. His views were partly based on the evidence from a survey of children with special needs in Camphill during the 1960s, which revealed, '...a strikingly higher percentage of first-born children among the psychotics' (Pietzner 1966, 213).

At that time, the term 'psychotic' was often used to describe children who might now be placed within the autistic spectrum. There is, however, no recent published evidence I am aware of to confirm these early observations.

Similarly, Weihs suggested that the numbers of children with autism who appear '...with large beautiful heads, and are potentially intelligent and gifted' (Weihs 1984, 90), were also more vulnerable, through their constitution, to the overpowering force of ego-awakening. As he had described in an earlier chapter of his book when speaking of large-headedness, 'Large-headedness is an expression of these children's own reluctance to be born' (Weihs 1984, 42).

It is interesting to note here that Kanner observed that of the eleven children with autism he originally saw, 'Five had relatively large heads' (1943, 248).

This 'reluctance to be born' as a longing to remain in a spiritual pre-birth existence can, in the case of some children with autism, be shown as an early lack of motivation with a weakened drive towards achieving ego-integration and the acceptance of personal karma.

Dr Hans Müller-Wiedemann

In the 1970s and early 1980s, Hans Müller-Wiedemann published his own attempts to try to come closer to a still more comprehensive and detailed anthroposophic understanding of autism. These were based on thirty years of practical experience living with children with autism. He also indicated some new perspectives in the areas of differentiated sensory developments.

Like König, he acknowledged the inability of children with autism to integrate themselves into the human environment via the power of imitation.

He also emphasised their fundamental inability to achieve an experience of their own body, and consequently to gain the inner security afforded by an existential, bodily-based self-experience.

He maintained that there was both an insufficient maturation and functioning of the lower senses and that, in fact, 'The extent of the "autistic disorder" depends, according to our experience, on the time-appropriate degrees of the development of the maturing of the lower senses' (Müller-Wiedemann *et al.* 1988, 69).

In particular, the sense of life, which normally develops during the infant's first year, is often severely disturbed. This had also been pointed out by König:

> We must only call to mind quite concretely what it means when the sense of life cannot develop as a contained uniform sense experience.
>
> If that happens then the child will not have a correct relationship to his own body. What is otherwise an immediate experience, starting in early childhood, by which we feel ourselves as being 'a complete within-ness' and thereby as a matter of course sense ourselves as a 'bodily self filling space'; this is not present.
>
> The identification between bodily corporeality and spirit-soul does not come about and thus severe contact disorders ensue. The child's soul experiences the body as

4. AUTISM SEEN ANTHROPOSOPHICALLY

not belonging to him, but rather as a part of the world. To a large extent the certainty of earth existence is thereby lost, and features and symptoms of severe autistic disorders appear. (König 1971, free translation by J. Holbek)

What König and Müller-Wiedemann both assert is vividly confirmed in the autobiography of a recovering person with autism:

My perception of a whole body was in bits. I was an arm or a leg or a nose. Sometimes one part would be very much there but the bit it was joined to felt as wooden as a table leg and just as dead. The only difference was the texture and the appearance. (Williams 1994, 228)

Furthermore, impairment of the sense of life would satisfactorily explain the often unusual and perplexing reactions of children with autism towards conditions that, in a normal child, would be the cause of severe pain or illness. For example, the self-injurious behaviours to which Wing refers (1996, 113).

The failure in the maturation of the lower senses does not allow a normal differentiation to develop between the body and the shared inter-human world of natural objects and other people. Consequently, as the process of individualisation of the body (towards the seventh year) is only partially achieved, facial expressions and movement patterns often remain almost unchanged up to the seventh year.

In terms of consciousness, it even appears that children with autism may become unhealthily awake in the perceptual realm of the lower senses, where they really ought to remain unconscious. This unusual awakeness is, for example, apparent in children being compulsively drawn into spatial-geometrical and mathematical relationships.

This appears in some children in the ritualistic ordering of objects. Elly Park (see Chapter 1) would, for example, arrange a hundred building blocks in perfectly parallel rows. A marked tendency to reduce the outer world to number and measure is seen, which is due to the pathological descent of consciousness into the lower sense realm: 'Everything which can be determined in our surroundings by number, measure and weight belongs to the experience realm of the four lower senses' (Aeppli 1993, 24).

This important realisation at once helps to explain the outstanding savant activities of some people with autism in the area of numbers and drawing (Wiltshire 1991). This led Müller-Wiedemann to write that, 'The child is "imprisoned" in the world of the lower senses which then also "invades" the field of the middle soul senses (Müller-Wiedemann *et al.* 1988, 75).

Children with autism do not awaken where they naturally should: in their head-centred thought life and self-consciousness. Therefore we can say children with autism have a certain reversal of normal consciousness. This significant insight was expressed by one anthroposophic researcher as follows:

> ...the autistic child as a whole assumes the character of a head, [but] the actual head itself is as though almost eliminated. The brain and the sense organs connected with it are restricted in their functions and altered.
> (Holtzapfel 1995, 42)

We can better understand Holtzapfel remarks when we realise that our nerve system is concentrated in the head (brain and senses). We use our senses and the brain to observe and reflect. This is a gesture of distance, of antipathy. Children with autism have this gesture of antipathy in their bodily nature: not wanting to be touched; keeping the environment the same instead of going with the flow; concentrating on mechanical objects instead of people. Their ability to speak, consciously observe and think is not so present. An example is a child with autism visiting the doctor. The child will flick the light switches, try the computer and the blood pressure machine and will not pay attention to the interaction, words or expression of the doctor. The child observes the doctors surgery through movement and actions.

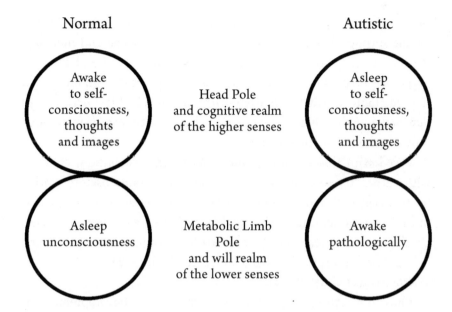

Figure 3. The reversal of consciousness in autism.

Moreover, the far-reaching seriousness of this reversal of conscious-ness for biography is highlighted when, from anthroposophy, we learn that our karmic intentions are embedded in the normally unconscious 'will' realm of the lower senses. Therefore, when children wake up pathologically into this realm, to a degree, they actually become con-scious of their karmic intentions, which can be a very real burden, causing pain and even acute despair (Müller-Wiedemann 1982). In Figure 3 the form of a lemniscate represents the two opposite poles of consciousness in the human being.

Furthermore, this reversed consciousness also prevents children with autism from attaining an inner world of living images and imagination. These images normally arise from early sensory-motor activities, since perceptual consciousness precedes the formation of such inner representations. The head remains empty because the normal mirroring faculty of the head and brain has been undermined.

The sense of thought, which is dependent on the healthy functioning of the sense of life, is also developmentally impaired. Since concepts cannot then be perceived, other sensory percepts, including those arising through language and gesture, lack both sense and meaning. It becomes clear that without enlightening concepts, the plethora of everyday percepts must present a confusing, painful, frightening and unpredictable world to children with autism. (In his *Philosophy of Spiritual Activity*, 1992, Steiner explains how reality is confirmed for us only when percept and concept unite together.)

Faced with this situation, and probably in desperation, children with autism try to create controlled and predictable pseudo worlds for themselves. Often children strive to maintain sameness at all costs, in order to reduce their existential fear: 'When we meet an autistic child it has to be clear to us that his world is not just deficient to ours, but that he creates for himself a world in which he can live' (Müller-Wiedemann *et al.* 1988, 66).

Only in a restricted space, without change and development, can they perhaps manage to gain some measure of inner security. However, if this space is breached, children are quickly filled with anxiety, fear and panic, as they immediately lose control over their environment. As Tustin (1992) expressed it, children with autism are often 'traumatised and terror-stricken'. These powerful emotions are certainly confirmed in the autobiographical accounts of Grandin (1986) and Williams (1992).

The senses and autism

The great importance Müller-Wiedemann attached to the under- or over-functioning of certain senses in autism is now recognised by mainstream literature (Delacato 1974; Ayres 1995). Delacato, for example, was convinced that for neurological reasons children with autism have an 'unreliable sensory system'. Disturbing experiences in autism due to abnormal sensory functioning and inadequate perceptual integration are confirmed in the autobiographical accounts of Grandin (1986) and Williams (1992 and 1994). Given the recent interest in and acceptance of the sensory aspect of autism, it is now clearly acknowledged in the DSM-5 (see Chapter 1). Therefore, the insights of anthroposophy were in many ways well ahead of their time. Due to the significance of the senses in autism, we have included a new chapter dedicated to this subject, with case studies from current social pedagogical practice (see Chapter 8).

Through anthroposophy's description of the twelve senses, and especially the relationships between them, we can begin to more fully understand the various possible sensory dysfunctions. In particular, we have pointed to the developmental relationships between the lower and the higher senses, such as the correspondence between the senses of touch and ego, and the senses of life and thought.

A classic example of the correspondence between tactile perceptions and an inner awareness of other people is vividly described by Temple Grandin (1986). By constructing a 'squeeze machine' for herself in order to experience whole-body pressure in a controlled way, she was able to first develop some empathy for others.

> At College I was making great strides in communicating
> with people. I attributed this 'break-through' in getting
> along better with people to my maligned squeeze
> machine. It enabled me to learn to be gentle, to have
> empathy... (Grandin 1986, 104)

We have suggested, and clearly predicted, the failure of certain higher senses, particularly those of thought and ego in children with autism. This prediction, if verified, would go a long way to explaining the so-called 'mind blindness', which Theory of Mind protagonists refer to (Frith 1989; Astington 1994). Theory of Mind refers to a person's natural ability to understand the connections between others' external behaviour and their inferred internal state of mind. This ability, which Frith (1989) calls 'mentalizing', is essential for us to function as socially aware human beings. In children with autism, this lack of mentalizing leads to a blindness regarding the minds of others.

We know that impairment in the functioning of the higher senses will have serious consequences for social communication, understanding and empathy. We also know that, as Müller-Wiedemann

(1966) described, it is precisely by the ego working in the child's social relationships that the whole realm of sensory perceptions can be properly assimilated and metamorphosed into meaningful personal experiences. However, this assimilation does not seem to happen in children with autism, so their perceptions lack coherent integration and meaningfulness. Therefore, Müller-Wiedemann seems convinced, as do I, that we find a fundamental problem of active ego-integration in these children. If the ego, the being of the child, is unable to properly take hold of its physical, etheric and astral bodies, and gradually penetrate and individualise them, sooner or later this will impact on both the organic and psychological levels, as current research into autism strongly suggests.

We could perhaps compare the complex process of typical ego-integration with the atypical autistic state in a very simplified way, as shown in Figure 4.

In a way, children with autism remain more closely connected to their pre-birth spiritual existence than normal children but, because of this, they do not develop sufficiently into the social-moral sphere. Müller-Wiedemann believes that this ego-integration difficulty has often arisen even before physical birth.

Primary causation

If the unborn child's soul-spiritual being (soul and spirit are united in pre-birth existence and also in young children) receives a shock, then the initial impulse and motivation towards the new incarnation may be seriously thwarted. Consequently, the crossing of the threshold between spiritual and earthly forms of existence will not be achieved successfully. Steiner gave indications that such an existential shock can occur, and thus prevent personal karma from being fulfilled. He described that, on the path of re-entry into physical life, the soul-spirit being experiences a pre-vision of its coming earthly life, and that, 'What he thus sees becomes the source of active forces which he must carry with him into the coming life' (Steiner 1989, 89).

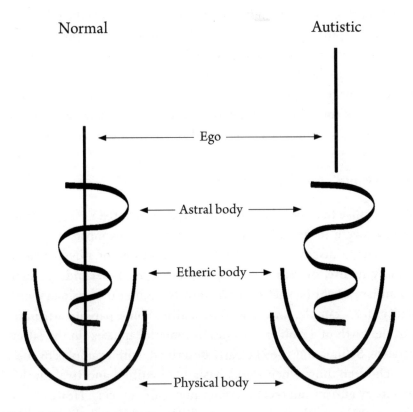

Normal   Autistic

Figure 4. *Typical ego-integration and autism.*

However, this pre-vision can sometimes be an overwhelming and threatening experience:

> Immediately before incarnation a very important event occurs, parallel to the event which follows the moment of death ... Not all the details are seen, but the circumstances of the coming life are made evident in broad outline. This is of the utmost importance. It may happen that a person who went through a great deal of suffering and hardship in his previous life receives a shock from the glimpse of the new circumstances and destiny now in prospect, and holds back the soul from complete incarnation. (Steiner 1970b, 49)

Rather than incarnate fully, the soul tries to remain in the pre-birth or pre-conceptual existence, and thereby to return to its spiritual past instead of turning its will impulse actively to the future. Such a reaction could, I suggest, be the original source for what then appears as a deep-seated and primary, early autistic condition, with a withdrawing from the sphere of social life. This sphere is, however, precisely the scenario where past karma must be encountered and new, future karma created.

Primary and secondary autisms

We recognise that there are different degrees of autism – a spectrum – from severe to mild. In terms of differential diagnosis it is very important to discover if the autism appears to be of a deep-seated primary nature, or rather of a secondary form. If secondary, then the autism could be due to a reaction to some other primary difficulty; for example, an early encephalitis. Some parents attribute it to the birth of a sibling, or a developmental aphasia. In the latter instance, Sahlmann (1969) clearly described, with examples of specific children, how when the aphasia is identified and treated, the secondary autism can recede, sometimes quite quickly. However, as Wing (1993) emphasised, accurate differential diagnosis can only be made by taking a detailed developmental history from infancy, and obtaining an equally detailed description of behaviour in different settings.

When the core symptoms of autism are present from childhood, it is likely that children will suffer some degree of autism for life unless, perhaps, we can begin to build trusting human relationships with them early on, through empathetic interventions based on a deepened understanding of their special existential predicament.

Asperger syndrome

The anthroposophic view of autism specifically relates to early infantile autism, as described and identified by Leo Kanner in 1943, which was historically referred to as Kanner's syndrome.

However, in 1944, Hans Asperger published a paper entitled 'Autistic psychopathy in childhood' (see Frith 1991, Chapter 2).

In recent years a great deal of interest has focused on gaining a better understanding of the nature of Asperger syndrome and its chief characteristics, as well as on distinguishing its similarities to and differences from Kanner's syndrome (Attwood 1998).

> Thus, to emphasise the differences, the young classic
> Kanner's child has good manual dexterity when
> engaged in his or her preferred activities but has delayed
> and deviant language development, as well as social
> impairment of the aloof kind. Those with typical Asperger
> syndrome have good grammatical speech from early in
> life, passive, odd or subtly inappropriate social interaction,
> and poor gross motor co-ordination shown in gait and
> posture. They also tend to be in the mildly retarded,
> normal or superior range of intelligence, while Kanner's
> group covers a wider range of the IQ scale ... However,
> the more able among Kanner's group can, over the years,
> develop the characteristics, including the types of social
> interaction, of people with Asperger syndrome, and
> become indistinguishable from them in adult life. (Frith
> 1991, 115)

What is, however, very clear is that children and young people with either of these syndromes show characteristic, often severe, difficulties with social interaction and integration. This can unfortunately lead to aloneness and isolation, and perhaps also acute frustration and despair in the comparatively more able person with Asperger syndrome.

Asperger Syndrome as a diagnosis will cease to exist after the introduction of the DSM-5 in May 2013 (see Chapter 1), but this does not negate the fact that children with autism, who can't speak or care for themselves, present very differently from intelligent, verbal but socially limited people with Asperger syndrome.

The anthroposophic interpretation of autism, as a fundamental problem of active ego-integration with insufficient individualisation of the child's three bodies (physical, etheric and astral), may need to be modified in order to explain Asperger syndrome. In children with autism we can quite easily imagine a certain withdrawal, and a consequent failure to achieve the typical incarnation process of soul and spirit into the body. However, it may be necessary with Asperger syndrome to speak of a too deep, or exaggerated incarnation process; perhaps a plunging down too strongly into earthly physicality. This would give rise to the characteristic clumsiness associated with Asperger syndrome, with a singular inflexibility of thought and complete lack of ordinary social understanding and empathy, in spite of often impressive language and intellectual abilities and specialised talents.

However, a detailed anthroposophic explanation of Asperger syndrome, and also any specific therapeutic exercises to alleviate it, would require further research work.

Self-consciousness and social life

We have come to understand that autism, whether primary or secondary, follows as the result of a child's reaction towards existential difficulties of incarnation. These difficulties can arise out of pre-earthly experience or possible hindrances found once incarnated in his or her body due to environmental factors. When this reaction occurs – before or soon after birth, or in the third year – will be crucial for the child's ongoing biographical development.

The very word *autism*, from the Greek word *autos* meaning *self*, strongly suggests that the child fails to achieve a normal process of earthly self-development, and therefore of successful ego-integration. Historically, with the fall from favour of psychodynamic approaches, and the increasing emphasis on behaviourism and organic causes of autism, the real significance of the meaning of the word autism, for the child's inner self-experience, has been eclipsed. As children with autism are unable, or perhaps sometimes unwilling, to come to the developmental experience of a secure and permanent self-consciousness, an active social life with truly interpersonal 'I'–'you' relationships is inevitably either absent or, at best, confused.

Some non-anthroposophic authors have also recognised the central significance of children's failure to achieve inner self-consciousness. For example, Hobson writes:

> The clinical vignettes [of earlier chapters] provide a rich source of insight into the children's relative lack of self-consciousness as well as their seeming obliviousness towards other people as 'selves' with their own interests, inclinations, motives, sensibilities, and so on. In addition, I have already linked autistic children's dearth of imitation with their lessened propensity to identify with the attitudes of other people. (Hobson 1993, 76)

Jordan and Powell also stress that, 'There is, in autism, a failure to develop satisfactorily an *experiencing self* (Jordan & Powell 1996).

As Leo Kanner originally described, this failure results in the typical outer appearance of 'extreme self-isolation, or aloneness'.

The challenge

These children are, however, not alone. It is very much our responsibility to discover ways to bridge the isolation created by an autistic reaction, and to build interpersonal relationships with these children. Autism is not merely an in-child problem, which perhaps has its roots in some form of brain damage or dysfunction. Anthroposophy views it as a special challenge to develop deepened, empathetic relationships with people who have encountered major difficulties on their path towards incarnation. To form such evolving relationships is indeed the foremost task of curative education, based on anthroposophy. It is of the greatest therapeutic importance to recognise that all children, whatever their behaviour, have real transcendent spiritual beings; this stands firmly at the heart of curative education (Hansmann 1992, 17). This clear and objective recognition of a child's true being can help to give the child's soul new forces of strength and courage with which to cross the threshold from the spiritual prenatal state to the human social world. We could say that each earthly life enables the individual to realise some part of his or her full human potential, precisely by facing up to life's challenges and obstacles.

III.

INTERVENTIONS AND ALLEVIATION

5. Some More Mainstream Interventions

Treatment or cure

According to the literature of recent decades, there is no known cure for autism (Schreibman 1988; Ellis 1990; Baron-Cohen & Bolton 1993; Happé 1994). In most cases it is a pervasive and life-long developmental disorder (Wing 1993; Trevarthen *et al.* 1996). Many children with autism never learn to speak during infancy, and remain mute. Unless children have acquired some useful, pragmatic speech by five years of age, their future prognosis is usually much less favourable in comparison to verbal children with autism (Aarons & Gittens 1992). Beyond childhood, and after adolescence and the demands of early adult life, there appears to be a tendency for any challenging behaviours to lessen, and for co-operativeness to increase (Wing 1990). However, irrespective of progress made or skills acquired, it appears that the vast majority of young people with autism continue to have social difficulties (Elliot 1990).

There are, it is true, isolated examples of remarkable recoveries from infantile autism (Kaufman 1976; Stehli 1991; Barron 1993). And there are stories of children who, according to their parents, reach a point where they no longer meet the criteria for a diagnosis of ASD, although such accounts are extremely rare. Reasons for this could be initial misdiagnosis, successful treatment, or even that some children grow out of certain forms of autism as they mature. I know one mother who told me her child no longer has the diagnosis of autism. And I recently read an account of a little girl called Kaylee who had been diagnosed with a 'moderate case of Autism Spectrum Disorder' at the age of sixteen months in the state of Illinois and, following antiviral and antifungal medication that addressed her immune system dysfunction, made a remarkable recovery:

> Three weeks after starting Valtrex (an antiviral medication) Kaylee looked into my eyes and called me 'Mom'. My heart swelled with joy because she had never addressed me as a person before. Kaylee started sleeping through the night and answering simple questions, every day slowly getting better and better. Then we addressed her allergies with a special treatment called P/N (otherwise known as Provocation/Neutralization), and her tantrums, hyperactivity, allergies, and food intolerances improved immediately.
>
> Over one year ago, Kaylee was re-tested by her school district and the result was that she no longer fit the diagnosis of Autism Spectrum Disorder. Today, Kaylee does not receive speech therapy, no longer has 'sensory' needs, and operates in a mainstream 1st grade classroom without an aide. Kaylee has friends, she has fun, and she's happy.
> ('Kaylee's Story of Recovery' www.treatingautism.co.uk)

There are some impressive autobiographical descriptions written by exceptional people with autism (Grandin 1986; Miedzianik 1986; Williams 1992, 1994).* Nevertheless, these outstanding successes are rare (Trevarthen *et al.* 1996). It challenges our viewpoint of autism as a medical and developmental condition when we hear from a vocal group who assert that autism is not an illness but a difference, which there is no need to cure. Some people with autism manage to live alone; they face challenges in daily life but feel no need to change.

Those people don't aim to become 'neurotypical', but point out that autistic thinking is different and can give new, innovative ideas, and that genetic research can become 'eugenics'. They find focus on community support, education and social services for people with autism more important thn finding explanations (Insel 2013).

* For a critical review of such autobiographical accounts see Happé in Frith (Ed.) 1991, 207–42.

Autism is still seen as a lifelong condition, but it is clear that many children and adults can be supported to develop and feel well in themselves and there are always remarkable stories about children who really change.

Education

In the 1960s, the importance of education for children with autism had already been recognised by some professionals. In 1967, Michael Rutter stated that, 'In our present state of knowledge education probably constitutes the most important aspect of treatment and it is to school in one form or another that we must look for the greatest hope of bringing about achievement in the autistic child' (Furneaux & Roberts 1979, 57).

Boucher and Scarth (1977) outline three different approaches to teaching children with autism:

1. The psychodynamic
2. Behaviour modification
3. Environmental

However, they point out that the structured, environmental approach, involving adult and task-directed activities, may also include elements of the more relationship-centred psychodynamic and/or the behaviourist methods. Since that time, the special learning difficulties shown by children with autism, and the development of different teaching methods and attitudes, have continued to be acknowledged and addressed (Elgar & Wing 1981; Jordan & Powell 1990 & 1996).

A particular behaviourist approach, developed by Erich Schopler, is known as the *TEACCH Program*. (TEACCH stands for Treatment and Education of Autistic and related Communication-handicapped CHildren.) It relies on a highly structured environment and individually-planned programmes of work (Sanderson & Fraley 1994).

Another behavioural intervention described by Rutter and Howlin (1989) recognised the need to involve the parents of children with autism as partners and participants in the implementation of home-based treatments.

However, in marked contrast to TEACCH and other behavioural methods, the Linwood Method for reaching 'the hidden child', has an emphasis on psychodynamic insights and interrelationships, in which, 'The focus is on educating the total child in an environment designed to make all experiences therapeutic' (Simons & Oishi 1987, 26).

Such a holistic educational and therapeutic approach is also practised in the Camphill and Steiner special schools, but there it is underpinned by anthroposophy's developmental Image of Man (Woodward 1985).

Other therapies and treatments

Research into autism is ongoing, but the quality and extent of research is still inadequate. Dr Hogenboom was a member of the NICE Guidelines group for autism for adults 2010–11, which found there was little new research available for adults with autism. Much of the information was of limited use because studies did not have enough participants, or research had to be extrapolated from learning disability groups. There is extensive research available regarding children with autism, but no groundbreaking new approaches have resulted from this.

The website for Research Autism (www.researchautism.net) collates all the latest available evidence regarding different interventions, and grades them according to suitability. It clearly indicates which interventions are currently recommended and which have been discredited. It is a valuable resource for parents or carers who may feel overwhelmed by all the possibilities. A selection of interventions are outlined and discussed below:

Auditory integration training (AIT) addresses the unusual, and often oversensitive, hearing perceptions of children with autism. The Berard Method employs systematic desensitisation or habituation of the child to particular, individually-assessed frequencies of sound that have been a source of distress. Another version of AIT, known as the Tomatis Method, aims to develop the active listening ability of children.

Berard's AIT received considerable impetus through the successful recovery from severe autism of Georgie, the daughter of Annabel Stehli (Stehli 1991). However, in common with other therapies that have relieved autism in some children, AIT still requires monitoring and controlled assessment to determine its efficacy for other children with autism (P & J Richardson 1994). AIT is not advised by the NICE Guidelines as treatment for autism.

Cognitive behavioural therapy (CBT) assumes that the way we think, feel and act are interrelated, and that by helping people become more aware of how they reason, they can change how they think and behave. Considerable research suggests that CBT can reduce anxiety in some people with autism, but it is only likely to work for higher-functioning people and older children, and can only be practised by appropriately trained therapists.

During *early intensive behavioural intervention* therapists break skills down into smaller, more achievable tasks. Desired behaviours, such as communication and social skills, are praised, whereas negative behaviours, such as self-harm and aggression, are discouraged.

Facilitated communication (FC) is a technique in which children with autism are given direct physical support by an adult facilitator, to either point to individual letters or words, or to type them on a keyboard. While the method is not claimed to be a cure for autism, its enthusiasts regard it as an important means of enabling communication. A book typed by means of FC, originally in German, described the profound experiences and inner conflicts of Birger Sellin, and received a lot of publicity (Sellin 1995; Holtzapfel 1993).

The book *Spiritual experiences of people with autism: Interviews with Hilke, Andreas, Erik and Martin Osika and Jos Meereboer*, edited by Wolfgang Weirauch, tells the story of three adults with non-speaking autism. These three brothers managed, through facilitated communication, to describe their difficult experiences in past lives, which meant they were not able to fully connect with their bodies in this life. One brother's memories go back to a Nazi concentration camp, one brother was tortured to death in order to betray the Jewish friends he hid, another was one of the guards. They explain that after such horrible experiences they did not want to come back to earth, but through meeting Christ they gained the courage to come as non-speaking people, so they wouldn't be faced with the same situations.

The major point of contention here is: who is actually doing the communicating – the person with autism or the facilitator? (Howlin 1994). Although such writings via FC can be impressive in content, one acclaimed American researcher recommends scepticism, 'It is now my considered opinion, after 35 years of experience [with FC] that what is being described as facilitated communication is invariably (unless proven otherwise) fraudulent' (Rimland 1996).

The NICE Guidelines for autism in adults 2012 officially state that FC should not be used, as there is insufficient evidence to prove that it is effective. There is, however, evidence that it can lead to harm; claims of sexual abuse have been made with FC, which were later not substantiated.

Incidental teaching takes into account children's own interests, using situations that arise naturally as the basis for teaching. For example, if a child shows an interest in a particular toy, the teacher might move it out of reach so the child has to communicate with the teacher in order to play with it. Incidental teaching has been used to teach various skills, including communication and social awareness. Similarly in *milieu training,* teaching is prompted by children's interest in an item or activity in the 'milieu' around them.

Intensive interaction (see Chapter 9 for a full exploration of this approach) was developed by Hewett & Nind (2000). It is a way of developing communication and building meaningful relationships with people with communication and severe learning difficulties. This is achieved by copying a child's behaviour and vocalisations with openness and interest, creating an atmosphere of exploration, with no dominance from the caregiver. One of the primary aims is to enjoy time together, so the child can learn that it's good to be with people.

Music therapy: children with autism are often very receptive to music, and therefore they can receive particular support and help through this medium. This has been clearly acknowledged in curative education, as well as in more mainstream therapies and research:

> Very severely autistic children who completely refuse
> to make use of language are often very musical and able
> to sing. Such children may sometimes be coaxed into a
> first kind of conversation on the basis of the duet. The
> therapist hums the first bars of a melody which the child
> may continue and thus, without looking at one another,
> they can sometimes establish a to and fro in a purely
> musical realm. (Weihs 1984, 96)

While such simple musical conversations may well be used by social pedagogues, it will additionally require the expertise of a music therapist to apply this field in a much more precise way, such that:

> ...melodies, intervals, single tones, pitch, harmony, rhythm
> and metre, are elements used therapeutically to work
> deeply into the living processes of specific organs and
> can aid ego-integration of a growing individual, as well as
> work on the emotional life. (Hansmann 1992, 138)

The Options (or Son-Rise) method, which was developed by Barry and Suzi Kaufman to help their son, Raun Kahlil, is an example of early, pre-school intervention. They started with this before he was two years old. At the core of the method is a complete acceptance of where the child is, and a willingness to try to enter into his autistic world. This might, for example, involve spinning objects with the child, perhaps for hours on end. 'We started to imitate him ... We wanted to use his cues as a basis of communicating' (Kaufman 1976, 62). The child's being is respected through this gentle, non-invasive attempt to build bridges of contact and communication.

By using the *picture exchange communication system (PECS)* children who can't talk or write can learn to communicate using pictures. Children are first taught to exchange a picture for an item they want. This can progress to using pictures to make whole sentences or communicate broader thoughts (see Chapters 9 and 10 for examples of this method in practice).

In *pivotal response training (PRT)* fundamental building blocks of child development, such as motivation, self-management, self-initiation and responding to multiple environmental cues are considered to be 'pivotal', because other behaviours, such as language, social interaction and challenging behaviour arise from them. This approach can be carried out in a naturalistic way by trained parents and carers.

Social Stories™ are a way of teaching social skills. Stories tailored to each child give explanations of difficult situations. They can be written down and illustrated or recorded. They have been used to lessen problematic behaviour and improve social skills in some children with autism.

Through *video modelling,* children with autism can learn by watching a recording of someone demonstrating a particular behaviour or skill, or individuals themselves can be recorded (video self modelling or VSM).

Visual schedules use a set of pictures to explain a series of activities or the sequence of steps in an activity, and can help some people with autism to understand future events.

Medication

Melatonin is a hormone and neurotransmitter that regulates our biological clock. In some people with autism it is not produced and used effectively, which can disrupt sleep and cause behavioural problems. Taking melatonin supplements can sometimes help.

Risperidone and *Olanzapine* are 'atypical antipsychotic' drugs, thought to alter the levels and activity of neurotransmitters in the brain, in particular serotonin and dopamine. Risperidone is used to treat aggression, self-harm and sudden mood swings; Olanzapine for hyperactivity, aggression and self-harm.

Conclusion

Intervening early is the most important thing to do, and this makes sense to all of us.

> We do know that significant improvement in autism symptoms is most often reported in connection with intensive early intervention ... and that many people with autism go on to live independent and fulfilling lives, and that *all* deserve the opportunity to work productively, develop meaningful and fulfilling relationships and enjoy life. With better interventions and supports available, those affected by autism are having better outcomes in all spheres of life. (Autism Speaks 2013b)

Looking at this list of approaches, it is clear that time and people intensive interactions support children with autism in their development. Visual approaches address the core issue of visual perception and integration, through PECS and video modelling, and these also prove to be helpful. Perhaps in fairness to all these contrasting interventions, we must admit that what may be helpful for one child may not work well for another.

In my experience with autism, parents have two choices: one group of parents works along with the professionals, taking early intervention and bringing their children to the local school with special support; the second group of parents starts the roller coaster of searching, and trying, every possible approach there is from dietary intervention, supplements, auditory training, tinted lenses, the Son-Rise approach and many more. They become 'professional' parents. All parents have to find their own way. The problem is that there is such a vast range of possibilities. The positive aspect of researching all the different approaches is engagement with, and hopefully improvement of, the child. The downfall can be social isolation of the child due to special diets, costs, energy and parents' time. Again, every child with autism is unique, and there is no single 'right' approach.

In the continued search for effective interventions there remains a pressing need to find a deepened and extended understanding of the real nature of this pervasive developmental disorder. In particular I will argue that the current, predominantly in-child (organic) view of autism is inadequate to meet the challenge of developing effective therapeutic relationships with these children. While we do have to accept that there is no known cure for autism, this does not mean that we cannot make significant strides towards its alleviation. A recent report in the *Guardian* suggested that many parents feel that good support, therapies and acceptance of autism are more realistic and important for them than looking for an elusive cure (Guardian readers & Ruth Spencer 2013). To improve support and treatment is, however, dependent upon the understanding we have towards children with autism. This in turn must be based on our understanding of human nature, and especially of early child development. Chapter 3 presents anthroposophy's holistic Image of Man as a foundation for seeing autism in a new light.

6. The Curative Educational Approach

The context for curative education

Until recently, the term 'curative education' was widely used to describe holistic educational centres, such as Camphill. It is a translation of *Heilpädagogik:* a word commonly used in German-speaking countries, which clearly links the educational process with a healing impulse: 'Curative education is that science which ... seeks predominantly pedagogical means for the treatment of intellectual and sensory defects, of nervous and emotional disturbances in children and adolescents' (Asperger 1956).

In its widest aspect, curative education is not only a science, not only a practical art, but also a human attitude.

> Only the help from man to man – the encounter of
> ego with ego – the becoming aware of the other man's
> individuality without enquiring into his creed, world
> conception or political affiliations, but simply the
> meeting, I to I, of two persons, creates that curative
> education which counters, in a healing way, the threat
> to our innermost humanity. This, however, can only be
> effective if with it a fundamental recognition is taken into
> consideration, a recognition which has to come out of the
> heart. (König in Pietzner 1990, 26)

This fundamental heart knowledge arises from the warmth of genuine interest, compassion and sympathy for the situation of the other human being.

The term 'social pedagogy' is now often used instead, due to the medical, diagnostic and school-based connotations of the term 'curative education', which were not always deemed appropriate. Both terms are still in use and are therefore both used in this book: chapters from the original edition and historical quotes mostly use the term 'curative education'; new chapters mostly use the term 'social pedagogy'. In the context of this book, both terms refer to practices informed by the values of anthroposophy.

Over the past 73 years, the Camphill organisation, or movement, has established therapeutic school and college communities, as well as village communities with adults (Pietzner 1990). There are more than one hundred Camphill communities in over twenty countries in Europe, North America, southern Africa and India. And curative education has been implemented in other anthroposophic residential and day centres for many years (Roggenkamp & Fischer 1974).

The aim is very much to keep children in their families and local communities, if possible. There are centres where experienced members of staff go out to families and support them in their own home. Other children benefit greatly from day placements, attending school every day but going home to sleep. Some children are weekly boarders, going home every weekend, and so still being integrated in their own family life.

There are still children who urgently need residential care: if they are not thriving in their school and local surroundings, and if the family has become exhausted and dominated by the overwhelming needs of a child. I remember many stories of children who would not sleep at home, and gradually learned to sleep once they settled into the rhythmical school lifestyle; or children with extremely restricted diets, who gradually broadened their diet by learning from other children at mealtimes.

In a therapeutic community such as a Camphill school, children with autism are integrated with other children with special needs, as well as with staff, children and adult co-workers, including experienced social pedagogues (teachers, house parents, therapists, doctors, etc.). Curative education, in this context, becomes a conscious way of life, which permeates equally the triad of home life, school and therapies.

Children with autism become members of their house community and their class of peers, as well as of the total community. The relationships between the different children are very important, and can often be a major therapeutic influence. For example, a sociable, outgoing child with Down's syndrome may be happy to include a withdrawn child with autism into some game or fantasy, without being at all put off or offended by their friend's autistic aloofness. The social and therapeutic value of educating children of mixed abilities, and with a variety of special needs, has always been acknowledged and practised in Camphill and other social pedagogical centres.

A rich cultural life, with the non-denominational celebrations of the main Christian festivals through music, art, drama, speech and song, is a common feature of all anthroposophic centres. For all children with special needs the rhythmic pattern of the year, colourfully marked by regularly recurring Christian festivals, becomes a familiar and culturally enlivened framework that supports their social existence. Meaning, purpose and clear structures permeate every aspect of life in a curative educational environment, and this, in turn, may help children with autism to experience a greater sense of meaning in their own lives (Hansmann 1992; Luxford 1994). Particularly the child's own sense of life, as an existential sensory experience, can be strengthened and fostered in a setting where daily, weekly and yearly rhythms are consciously cultivated to create a healthy way of life. It is in such a holistic and thoroughly human context that special curative educational interventions and exercises can best be practised.

> Therefore it can also, in the education of autistic children,
> be considered to be the most important aim – besides all
> special measures – to enable these children to live as people,
> as free as possible, albeit with difficulties, with other people
> in community. (Müller-Wiedemann *et al.* 1988, 182)

Anthroposophic interventions

The following interventions are all compatible with the anthroposophic model presented in Chapters 3 and 4, and are strongly suggested, or generated, by that model. We can summarise these intervention areas as:

1. Inter-human attitudes
2. Imitation, rhythmic activities and play
3. Sensory-perceptual development
4. School curriculum
5. Crafts and work
6. Specific therapies and medical treatments

Inter-human attitudes

The power of empathy must be the foundation of all genuine (also non-anthroposophic) intervention attempts. This power can be developed by educators, whether they are teachers, house parents or therapists. Steiner indicated precisely how this could be done when, in the second of the twelve lectures on curative education, he described the Pedagogical Law, which intimately links both educator and child (Steiner 1972, 39). This fundamental relationship is indicated in Table 4.

Educator ⟶	Child
Ego	Astral Body
Astral Body	Etheric Body
Etheric Body	Physical Body

Table 4. The inner relationship between educator and child.

This means that the educator's ego has a direct influence on the astral body of the child, their astral body on the child's etheric body, and their etheric body on the child's physical body. Steiner indicated how educators must be willing to consciously develop and work upon their own being and bodily sheaths in order to bring healthy and vitalising influences to the child's bodily constitution. For example, 'By ridding himself of every trace of subjective reaction the teacher educates his own astral body' (Steiner 1972, 40).

This is then able to extend positive and corrective effects on a child's inner etheric organisation.

Following a moral path of self-development and genuine self-knowledge was considered by Steiner to be essential for a curative teacher: 'For you have no idea how unimportant is all that the teacher says or does not say on the surface, and how important what he himself is, as teacher' (Steiner 1972, 41).

Therefore we see that developing human interrelationships consciously, informed by anthroposophy's differentiated Image of Man, is at the heart of curative education. It is necessary to build up a relationship that engenders mutual trust and confidence. A child with autism is in many ways insecure and anxious, and possibly, at times, terrified. Since the child has not yet achieved a centred self-consciousness, an indirect, non-invasive approach should generally be adopted.

> This therapeutic attitude entails never confronting the
> child directly. We should never attempt to look into his
> eyes and address him as we would another person. Rather
> it is necessary to learn to see that the autistic child is not
> truly 'in himself', and that we can reach him if we address
> ourselves to his 'peripheral self', to that which is not
> centred. (Weihs 1984, 92)

This indirect attitude is the opposite of the confrontational approach of Holding Therapy, developed by Martha Welch, in which mothers are advised to face and forcefully hold children with autism. We often deliberately leave a *space* for children to enter into when they feel able and ready to do so. This space can be a *soul* space, created through

113

our empathy, and sometimes also a *physical* space. Some children with autism react with distress if expected to enter a room with many other people, such as a dining room. However, the same children may manage well if allowed to go into an empty room first and then be joined by others.

Again, the opportunity to be outdoors, in wide natural surroundings, can often provide observable relief for such children. As a general rule, genuine enthusiasm should not lead an educator to be over-demanding or to ask too much of children with autism. Compulsive and ritualistic behaviours may largely be accepted and allowed, provided that they do not seriously interfere with others. If children feel properly understood and accepted, such behaviours may relax or even disappear of their own accord.

Imitation, rhythmic activities and play

These three areas are interrelated and can support each other. In the 1960s, König was clear that in order to help children with autism, they need to learn to imitate and play (König 1960 & 1989). How to do this of course depends on the individual child and the creativity of the educator.

Normally, young children naturally imitate what is going on in their surroundings, including the work of adults. However, as this usually does not come about spontaneously with children with autism, the imitation of actions needs to be taught as a conscious intervention. This can include rhythmic to and fro activities, turn-taking activities and simple play. For example, when building a tower with toy bricks, adults can first show children how it is done, and then try to engage them one brick at a time. This can be accompanied by simple speech, 'I place a brick, you place a brick,' and so on. Starting perhaps from sitting behind the child, the adult can then sit next to, and finally opposite the child.

Depending on the age of the child, a variety of games can also be used to establish interrelationships.

> These can be ball or ring games, or simple dances
> connected with songs and rhymes. For children not
> ready to enter into a game situation, however, simple
> clapping exercises between child and therapist, crosswise
> and parallel, can be helpful, or even more rudimentary
> measures, such as infant games with fingers and toes.
> (Weihs 1984, 95)

It may be quite possible to slowly involve children with autism in traditional ring games with a group of peers, in which the children first stand, take hands and form a circle (Opie 1988). Children who will not initially join in may do so in time if a space is left for them to enter into, when they themselves feel able and ready to join. Singing and ring games, such as, 'Here we Go Round the Mulberry Bush'; 'Water, Water Wallflower' and 'Poor Jenny a-Weeping', have definite therapeutic benefits, which can help children to develop their learning abilities and also their self and social awareness (Heider 1995).

Eurythmy movements corresponding to the sounds of speech can also be done on an individual basis or with others (Raffe *et al.* 1974; Steiner 1967). If children are first physically helped to perform such gestures from behind, they may, through their own sense of movement, begin to experience some joy in the gestures and eventually start to imitate them spontaneously.

Play with various materials such as sand, water, beeswax, clay or other objects can be fostered as a reciprocal activity between adult and child, and perhaps later with peers. By doing so children's repetitive, bizarre or ritualised behaviours can be led into the inter-human realm.

Sensory-perceptual development

As the anthroposophic model emphasises, the proper functioning of children's four lower senses is of existential importance. It also provides the foundation for the proper development of the higher, social senses. Müller-Wiedemann (1990) has shown that disorders of the lower, or body senses often appear as:

1. A disturbed relationship with organic substances, with nutritional and digestive problems (sense of life).
2. Stereotypic and bizarre movement patterns (sense of movement).
3. The avoidance of experiences and exploration through touch and, often, in the child's inappropriate touching of others (sense of touch).
4. In the realm of gravity, a compulsive dependency on spatial positioning: walking on tiptoes, making roundabout turns, spinning of objects or own body, placid muscle tone (sense of balance).

It is interesting to note that children with autism often appear to be very able in terms of balance and movement. However, as Engel (1968) described, both exceptional abilities in these areas and abnormal movement patterns can be understood as the lack of ego-integration within these two lower senses, and the resulting preponderance of instinctive, astral soul activity.

Some curative educational interventions directed to the lower senses are given below. All such interventions aim to stimulate the child's own motivation and, through this, to individualise the field of the lower senses. The senses of hearing and warmth will also be considered here, with examples of some of the interventions described by Müller-Wiedemann (1990).

SENSE OF LIFE

Over the course of time, children can learn to accept varied foods in regular daily meals, when only small portions of the foods they have an aversion to are given initially (children with autism often have compulsive food fads). Care may be needed to provide an eating environment where other sensory impressions are reduced – a peaceful instead of a noisy dining room, mellow lighting etc.

A rhythmic pattern and predictability in children's daily life is particularly significant for developing the sense of life. This is consciously created in holistic community living in Camphill and other centres and, through this, children with autism are embedded and supported by definite life rhythms. We have already emphasised the special disturbance of the sense of life in children with autism (see Chapter 4). Their often unusual reactions to circumstances that would normally cause bodily pain, sometimes even severe pain, can be clearly understood as a direct symptom of the immature development of this sense.

Children are helped to better perceive their state of bodily health through nutritional and rhythmic interventions such as those described above. Anthroposophic medicines and special baths can also help to stimulate and order the metabolic processes (see also 'Sense of warmth' and Chapters 14 and 15).

SENSE OF MOVEMENT

Although eurythmy movements have special value here, all forms of co-ordinated movement exercises can be attempted and practised. Müller-Wiedemann (1982) recommended that children be helped to make slow movements, as children with autism tend to do things quickly as if they have no time. Again, many children show a tendency towards symmetry. Here, laterality and dominance exercises are important, such as catching and throwing a rod with the dominant hand. With older pupils aim exercises with a bow and arrow, or fencing, have proved helpful (Weihs 1984).

Form or dynamic drawing, applied therapeutically, stimulates ego-integration and bodily self-experience through the sense of movement, and also through the senses of balance and life (Niederhäuser & Frohlich 1974; Kirchner 1977). Such exercises involving the rhythmical drawing of curved or straight-line forms have been used helpfully with some children with autism. Forms that require children to cross over lines, when drawing lemniscates for example, can help to strengthen their inner self-awareness.

SENSE OF TOUCH

This can be developed by activities in which children are helped to discriminate between the feel of contrasting surfaces and objects. First, the educator takes the initiative to stimulate the child's tactile perceptions, for example, by touching exposed skin areas such as the face, neck, arms, lower legs and feet with a variety of materials. Brushes of different textures can also be used effectively. Later, children can be led into explorative touching, also without visual input if objects are hidden in sand or beneath a cloth. Importantly, children can be guided to touch, identify and explore their own bodies. Clearly the aim of such exercises is to establish children's own body boundaries – and thereby their self-experience – with regard to the surroundings. Both the separation and distance between *self* and *world* is thereby strengthened.

SENSE OF BALANCE

This sense is stimulated by children coming to terms with the force of gravity through resistance exercises, and by experiencing weight. For example, children with autism are asked and shown how to carry heavy objects across a room. This can be performed as a turn-taking exercise with the educator/therapist. Medicine-ball games, exercises with hand weights, balancing, walking with lead-weighted anklets in order to enhance the experience of gravity, and partner resistance exercises can be used.

Success with lower sense exercises can be clearly indicated by increased eye contact, social smiling, a lessening of obsessional behaviours, greater relaxation, increased muscle tone, a widened diet and improved sleeping-waking patterns. In effect, these are all indicators of better ego-integration.

Children with autism are often overwhelmed by meaningless percepts, and are unable to integrate them into coherent personal experiences. Therefore, in general, care must be taken to protect children from too much sensory stimulation and exposure. Without this care, children can only withdraw, perhaps into ritualistic behaviours, as a form of defence strategy.

SENSE OF HEARING

Curative educational interventions that develop an active use of the sense of hearing (the first of the higher social senses) aim especially to increase children's listening capacities. Exercises are done to further, or newly develop, the connection between listening and movement organisation; that is, muscle tone as the basis of perceptional interest and the processing of auditory percepts (see Appendix 1). The stereotypic fixation of a child's movements, and also slack muscle tone, are both outer signs of insufficient sensory ego-integration. They can lead to a high degree of avoidance within the acoustic realm, including speech, and sometimes appear as an oversensitivity to certain tones or sounds. Therefore, interventions that involve both movement and listening are used: such as tone eurythmy, in which children are guided to make specific eurythmy gestures corresponding to specific heard tones.

Improvised musical conversations, where the therapist speaks to children with tone phrases on a lyre and the children are encouraged to answer freely on their lyre, also provide a means of communication. Such tone conversations have the power to undo some children's tendency to talk to themselves, which can become a pathological habit, preventing spontaneous communication due to the preponderance of rigid memories. As such, the value of music for children with autism has long been acknowledged (Weihs 1984; Alvin & Warwick 1992). Some of these musical interventions take the form of specialised therapies.

SENSE OF WARMTH

This middle or 'soul sense' has a quite particular significance in the *twelvefoldness* of the sensory organism (see Appendix 1): 'It is the archetypal sense, which has a primary presence in all other senses' (Soesman 1990, 97).

In terms of the human soul, it enables a warm interest and responsiveness to take place between child and world, including the social world. Some children with autism show hyposensitive reactions to both heat and cold.

Pyrogenic baths, in which the temperature is raised by one or two degrees centigrade above the usual body temperature, have been used successfully for children with autism (see also Chapters 14 and 15). According to Müller-Wiedemann, 'During and after such applications the children make better eye contact; in speaking children, their speech is activated, and one can better communicate with simple games and with imitation' (Müller-Wiedemann 1990).

Similar positive effects also result from using warm foot baths in the morning and then rubbing until the feet become pink. Foot baths given in the evening can help children go to sleep. Through warmth interventions of this kind, ego-integration is facilitated and soul expression and responsiveness stimulated. It should, however, be emphasised that therapeutic measures such as pyrogenic baths require the recommendation of a qualified medical practitioner, as well as the expertise of trained curative educators.

School curriculum

In curative education the use of the Steiner-Waldorf school curriculum has a major role to play (Woodward 1985; Hansmann 1992). However, the effectiveness of the curriculum, both for children with autism and with other special needs, depends centrally on the empathetic relationships developed by teachers with their classes and individual pupils (Weihs 1975, 103). Both in mainstream Steiner-Waldorf schools and in curative schools, having the same class teacher – ideally from the ages of six to fourteen – is of unique importance. This allows time for relationships to grow and mature, and is also a challenge for the educator's path of self-knowledge.

The Steiner-Waldorf curriculum, which was outlined by Steiner in his many educational lecture cycles, is based on the anthropo-sophic understanding of child development, and the typical stages of ego-integration. When this is applied pedagogically to a class of children with special needs and diverse abilities, as has been practised for more than sixty years in Camphill schools, it is found that, 'The Waldorf syllabus, as part of our overall curriculum, furthers and restores harmony between body, mind and spirit, and is the strongest educational healing element we can apply' (Hansmann 1992, 83).

When one or more children with autism are integrated socially with their peers into a class, and taught according to the Steiner-Waldorf curriculum, they are fully recognised and respected as human beings in the process of becoming. The age appropriateness of the subjects and activities in the curriculum always aim to foster the sense of dignity and self-esteem in each child. As one curative school expressed it, 'The Steiner-Waldorf curriculum, adapted to the child's ability to understand, is one of the most powerful tools to help autistic people to find themselves and their place in the world.'

Even if children with autism do not outwardly appear to be taking in much of what is brought to the class, it is an unjustified assumption to think that they are not aware of what is happening. The inner attitude of teachers, and their awareness of the child's being, is of prime importance in what are often very subtle processes of interaction. With children with autism, where an indirect approach is usually called for, their peripheric consciousness and sensitivity to their surroundings must be acknowledged. The clear form, structure and predictability of much of the school day and week provide important support to children with autism.

Crafts and work

For children with autism, and more particularly for adolescents, these two areas of learning can often be of very great help and support. Crafts, which are also an essential part of the Steiner-Waldorf curriculum, can include weaving, basketry, woodwork, pottery, candle making, metalwork and bookbinding. Work can take the form of helping with daily household tasks, such as sweeping the floor, laying the table, or washing- and drying-up, etc. Land work and gardening have often

121

proved effective with older pupils, especially heavy tasks such as pushing a loaded wheelbarrow. Log sawing provides a good, rhythmic and interactive activity with a partner.

The variety of craft and work activities belong in the sphere of holistic education, in which the growing relationships and attitudes between educator and pupils are central. Through these interactions, and the educator's empathetic attitudes, even a mundane daily task such as drying the dishes can become a valuable therapeutic exercise. Often such tasks also serve as a medium for social integration, communication and gradual participation with others. Writing on the theme of youth guidance in curative education, Luxford remarks that:

> Craft work and other kinds of practical activities should play a larger part in the education of the youngster and particularly that of the student with special needs. A new area of self-recognition can be gained in the encounter with craft and practical activities. Crafts are particularly important because through these, skill training, observation, judgments and social motivation unite in the forming of a bowl, the weaving of a basket, or the dipping of a candle. (Luxford 1994, 97)

From my own experience, weaving has proved to be of particular benefit for adolescents with autism, who seem to find security, order and peace in this essentially rhythmic activity, and communication and conversation can sometimes occur whilst the youngster weaves.

Work and crafts that have clearly visible end results can help to provide meaning and sense to people with autism. This can be witnessed particularly in the purposeful integration of adults in the life of sheltered village communities (Farrants 1988; Pietzner 1990; Christie 1989; Frankland 1995).

Specific therapies

These particular interventions are prescribed on a purely individual basis during the internal reviews or clinics held for pupils in the school or centre they attend, and the centre's anthroposophic medical adviser is always present. Clinics take place once or twice a year for each child, though they can be called more often if needed.

Specific therapies require the expertise of curative educators who have received some training in the particular therapy concerned. However, as with the lower sense exercises described earlier in this chapter, they do not necessarily require a specially qualified therapist.

As there is no one therapy for autism, it is always necessary to see which therapy can best meet an individual child's needs at that time, from the range of therapies available in the centre that have proved helpful for other children with autism (Hansmann 1992; Müller-Wiedemann 1990; Weihs 1984). Ideally a specific therapy will take place three (or more) times a week, and continue for at least several months. Again it must be emphasised that the interrelationships between therapist and child are of key importance. Anthroposophic therapists will realise that they are also continually learning and developing, through the acknowledgment of the child's spiritual-soul being and their special situation in the world. The work must always involve a dynamic, two-way process on a number of different, but connected, levels of involvement.

ART THERAPY

Art therapists will usually be able to offer painting, modelling and drawing to meet the child's needs. The therapy, in whichever medium, aims to harmonise the threefold nature of the child (see Chapter 3), by working especially on the rhythmic system and the feeling life. By strengthening this middle sphere of breathing and blood circulation, a dynamic balance can be developed within the human threefoldness, both for body and soul.

Painting, for example, makes use of the differential qualities of

123

colours, and their relationships and gestures (Hauschka 1985). Painting and colours work particularly on the child's astral nature. Modelling strengthens the etheric body. Form or dynamic drawing stimulates the lower senses. Ego-integration through the middle senses of sight, warmth, smell and taste, can be cultivated through anthroposophic art therapy, and children with autism can benefit greatly from this, when using the medium best suited to meet their individual needs (see also Chapter 10 for an example of art being used in a therapeutic setting).

EURYTHMY THERAPY

Of all the therapies in the field of social pedagogy, this is probably the most important. It must be applied by a trained eurythmy therapist working under the advice of an anthroposophic doctor, and done with each child individually. Special eurythmy movements, based on speech sounds and musical tones, are used according to the individual diagnosis. These movements work deeply into the etheric formative forces and organs in the child's body (Kirchner-Bockholt 1992). When prescribed for a particular child with autism, the therapist first needs to gain the child's trust and co-operation, in order to lead them into active participation in the exercises.

PLAY THERAPY

Children with autism have little or no ability to play creatively or spontaneously. Therefore this therapy, guided by the therapist's empathetic understanding, can be especially helpful: 'The child can be led from a set, inflexible way of being, into a future with new possibilities of expression and experience' (Hansmann 1992, 146).

Therapists are called upon to create an inner soul space within themselves, which can receive and accept children as they are, and also recognise the difficulties that confront children's real being. This inter-relationship with children calls upon the therapist's own creative and imaginative potential, and can employ a wide range of materials. *Dibs in search of self,* by Virginia Axline, gives a moving and classic account of the value of play therapy in psychotherapy with an emotionally withdrawn child.

While not confined to play therapy, the use of a puppet theatre for children with autism can be included here. The very indirectness and non-commitment involved with a puppet show can bring relief and pleasure.

> The most severely withdrawn child will become
> indistinguishable from other normal healthy children in
> his reaction to a puppet performance, for he can enjoy and
> participate in a great variety of dramatic human situations
> without committing himself. (Weihs 1984, 97)

RHYTHMICAL MASSAGE

Massage must be rhythmical in order to strengthen the forces of the rhythmic middle system in the human threefoldness, which especially supports the feeling life of the soul (Evans & Rodger 2000). Moreover, it is through breathing that the incarnation process takes place. Therefore this therapy can also be used to help a child with autism to achieve better ego-integration, provided the child will tolerate direct touching. In this massage treatment special oils are used, as indicated by the doctor, to enhance the therapeutic effects.

Medical treatments

The use of anthroposophic, potentised remedies and medicines is very important in the totality of curative education, and is clearly the prerogative of a qualified doctor. However, the doctor's diagnosis and subsequent treatments are arrived at partly by listening to the descriptions given in review meetings by curative educators who know the children well. Treatment must be based on a thorough knowledge of the fourfold human constitution and the threefold organic systems (see Chapter 3). The doctor's insights and observations help the educator to see exactly how these are related and functioning in a particular child.

125

Anthroposophic medicines aim to treat or remedy the illness or disorder, and not merely eliminate symptoms. The specific therapies discussed above should be viewed as an integral part of holistic treatments for, and with, children with autism.

The college meeting

Interpersonal, interdependent relationships and empathy are at the centre of curative education. These are highlighted when a college meeting is held in a school community. This special meeting is centred on a particular child, and all the educators who teach, live and work with that child are present. Through listening to an account of the child's early history and their progress and difficulties since coming to the centre, they endeavour to gain a deeper insight into and recognition of the child's being, and perhaps something of the child's personal karma.

Although children are not physically present at this event, a college meeting can help to positively change and develop the interrelationships between children and their educators through a new anthroposophic understanding of their situation. However, for developmental reasons and out of respect for the individual's dignity and freedom, a college meeting is not usually held for pupils over the age of fourteen.

Autism should not merely be seen as an in-child problem, as it appears when viewed on the purely organic level of causation. Rather it should be viewed as a challenge to our own willingness to build genuine human relationships, despite the difficulties autistic reactions present us with. The college meeting is therefore an important and central intervention event in curative education.

7. A Curative Education Case Study: James

BOB WOODWARD

In this section we shall look at the development of my interrelationships with a boy with autism, together with the implementation of specific interventions and curative attitudes. I worked with two boys, who were residential pupils in a Camphill community school, but details of just one case study have been included in this revised edition. The anthroposophic model of autism gives the clear, underlying basis for all of this, and it is important to keep in mind the holistic context for curative education, described at the beginning of Chapter 6. There are many differentiated areas for positive interventions, through which children with autism can gradually integrate into the triad of home life, school and therapies, and become members of the school community. As I am not trained as a specialist therapist (such as a eurythmy or art therapist), the therapeutic measures I practised with the boys were derived from the first three intervention areas, described at length in Chapter 6:

1. Inter-human attitudes
2. Imitation, rhythmic activities and play
3. Sensory-perceptual development

This interventional work was a further continuation of research I had already been engaged in for several years.

My goal was to develop the interrelationship between myself and the boy, and to develop and implement an individual programme of exercises in order to alleviate the autism. Each session involved a continuous process of observation and assessment of how we were responding and reacting with each other. I considered my own inner attitudes, thoughts and feelings to be an integral part of the therapeutic situation and process, as well as the child's behaviours and actions. The evaluation process involved observations from others in the school community and the child's parents, as well as my own.

James: a brief background

The information given below over the crucial first three years was derived from the boy's case files: from recordings of interviews that took place prior to him being admitted to Camphill community school, and from his educational, psychological and medical records.

Features of early development

James was a third child to a 26-year-old mother, conceived six months after the birth of his sister. Although the child was planned, the mother felt unhappy throughout her pregnancy. Otherwise the pregnancy was normal except for slightly raised blood pressure and an unspecified fall or blow at full term.

Labour took five hours, and the birth was described as easy and difficult! James did not cry at once and was jaundiced for three days. He had a very low APGAR score at birth and was given oxygen.

James was a restless baby, quite 'whingy', and didn't show affection to or look at his mother. He smiled late. At one and a half months he was admitted to hospital for observation for a cough and had his first immunisation (not whooping cough). He was breastfed for four to five months, fed well and gained weight. He sat unaided at seven months but never crawled. Teething started at ten months.

At sixteen months his mother encouraged him to walk by standing him against the wall. And at eighteen months he walked by himself. Aged twenty months, he did not point, did not look at people. He lined up his toys, showing repetitive patterns of behaviour. There was no speech development; he did not respond to noise, sounds or voices.

During his first year James still did not speak and was diagnosed as 'a little boy with autism'.

James' mother informed me that James was 'freezing cold' when he was born in the middle of the night in the summer. His skin looked almost 'black' and he just 'hung'. Altogether his appearance at birth was 'a great shock'. Seemingly, James did speak a few single words at around thirty months, but without any further progress.

She described James as a 'restless baby'; later he became a 'very placid child', who became more affectionate with his close family. He tolerated other children, but did not interact with them. As a young child he was prone to viruses and was seen by an ear, nose and throat (ENT) special-ist and fitted with grommets. He also saw an eye specialist for his squint. According to his mother, James had various tests – 'too many to remem-ber' – and was seen by 'lots of psychologists' over the years. A psychologi-cal update when he was seven years old described him as, 'a profoundly autistic little boy whose difficulties in learning are severe and complex.'

James attended a special unit in a mainstream day school for four years. Aged five and six, he was said to have 'poor bodily awareness'. When he was eight years old he came to his present Camphill community school as a termly residential pupil who was not yet toilet-trained. The school's medical adviser confirmed James' diagnosis as a 'deeply autistic boy'.

Finally, and perhaps significantly, it should be noted that his mother commented, 'I have also thought that James somewhere along the line made a choice not to speak (if that doesn't sound a bit strange).' Whether or not James did make such a choice, we should always take such intuitive impressions seriously, as a mother has a special connection towards the real being of her child.

Diagnosis

James had received a definite diagnosis of autism and had shown autistic symptoms within the first three years of life. He had been jaundiced for three days after birth, had required some special treatment (oxygen) and was prone to viruses from an early age.

It seems possible that, with his early health problems, low APGAR score and ENT investigations, James' autism might have been a secondary reaction to other primary difficulties. In James' case, there has been no sign of any speech development up to the present day. Interestingly, he has a largish head, as did five of Kanner's original sample of eleven children (see Chapter 4).

Principles of the interventions

As mentioned earlier, the three areas from which I designed an individual programme of intervention were: 1. Inter-human attitudes; 2. Imitation, rhythmic activities and play; 3. Sensory-perceptual development.

Within the third of these areas the realm of the lower senses was specifically addressed, in order to facilitate the process of ego-integration, and the increased use of the child's higher social senses for interpersonal contact and communication. As we have seen, a fundamental principle of all anthroposophic interventions is that of mutual changes and developments in both pupil and educator. Participants are therefore interdependent. This principle acknowledges that the degree of autism is not only an in-child condition but also, and possibly equally, an environmental issue.

Procedure and implementation

The individual sessions took place between September 1998 and March 1999. James went home for a two-week half-term holiday in the autumn, three weeks at Christmas and a week in the spring. One special feature of the work was the increased frequency of the interventional input: around forty minutes, four times a week during the autumn term, and three times a week during the spring term; I carried out 59 sessions, with a single, sixtieth follow-up session in the summer term.

Each session took place in the same physical surroundings, the school's large movement hall, and at the same time in the morning, thus providing a predictable and consistent rhythm to each school week.

The second special feature of my work with James was that no other therapies or remedies were given during the period of my interventions, so it was considered likely that any significant changes (for better or worse) could be attributed to my sessions, over and above any natural developmental factors.

The third special feature was that the programme was flexible and had been derived from observing the child's responses when first trying out activities together. The actual implementation called for some give and take by both of us, as joint participants in a therapeutic process. At times, for example, I could be firmer in my expectations towards James and, depending on his state of health and openness, at other times more flexible and amenable to his wishes; much depended on feeling my way through each session and learning together.

Developing a relationship

I had already worked with James in September 1997, before starting these more frequent sessions. He had only just been admitted to the school, and was eight years and three months old. At that time, we worked in the playroom and I tried to engage his interest in a variety of activities that particularly called upon his lower senses of touch, balance and movement.

During that earlier intervention period I felt that we had gradually developed a therapeutic relationship, built on mutual trust and confidence. James became more actively co-operative in the exercises we did, also responding well to hands-on physical contact, such as tickling, but he made very little eye contact and appeared to deliberately avoid it. I worked with him and adapted my expectations and hopes in the light of his reactions and responses, rather than forcing the issue.

James had no speech, and often made rather anxious-sounding noises. He also showed obsessive, apparently meaningless behaviours, such as manipulating toy building bricks in his fingers.

Progress was made over these original nineteen sessions in building our relationship, getting to know each other, and by encouraging James to engage in various joint activities. At times he became more open,

131

and interpersonal contact then increased; for example, when tickling or teasing him, or when imitating his noises. There were also moments when he looked towards me and smiled, occasionally making brief eye contact and becoming quiet and peaceful; for example, when touching different surfaces.

These early sessions serve as an example of the progress James made in engaging himself in a meaningful, co-ordinated activity with attention and dexterity. In the first session, James had not shown the slightest interest in building a tower with bricks. After working patiently on this together, and as a turn-taking exercise, by the eighteenth session I recorded, 'Today he built a tower more or less by himself! In this activity he is attentive, and shows good dexterity.' He thereafter continued to demonstrate his tower-building skills back in his classroom.

By September 1998, when I resumed my therapeutic relationship to James, he was nine years old, and had settled down well during his first year at the school. He was still not toilet-trained and therefore wore disposable nappies.

First half of the autumn term, 1998

Session 1: 3 September, 1998

We went for the first time into the movement hall. James was not very happy about that to begin with.

I tried to have some interaction with him using a beanbag and a ball. He screwed up the beanbag in his hands. Didn't hand it back to me. I took it and put it on his head a number of times, in a rather playful way. I ran up and down the movement hall with James a number of times. He went along with this. I also held his hands and swung him around (but not off the floor). He seemed to enjoy this.

Then I got out the big gym mattress. He showed a real interest in this, for bouncing on. Also he lay down on it, or rather I laid him down on it, and rolled him over – which he obviously enjoyed.

He participated in, and generally enjoyed, these gross movement activities – running, swinging round, bouncing, rolling.

James did make eye contact at various times. He also came and took me by the arm or hand when he wanted me to go with him (e.g. to the mattress). When he didn't want to go with me he would grip or pinch.

He hyperventilates quite a bit. Makes noises; no words or clear sounds. His hands were firm, lean, bony, dry (not particularly warm or cold I think). He is a thin, lean-looking boy, with a largish-looking broad head and a wide mouth.

So today I experienced that: he can pull strongly when he wants to go somewhere; he can whine and protest when he wants his way. He also appears to enjoy various gross movements, and to clearly indicate that he wants more of this, particularly so with bouncing on the mattress.

On the basis of these initial experiences with James, the subsequent sessions consisted largely of gross movement and balancing activities, which included:

- Walking along and stepping over benches.
- Stepping onto a chair, and jumping down from it.
- Carrying weighted shopping bags, containing large stones.
- Climbing up and down wall bars.
- Walking with James, as he stood on my feet and I held his upper body.

In all these exercises, which called upon James' lower senses, I carefully observed his responses and was open to inspiration as to what to do next. This led to the introduction of touch activities in the fifth session and to *body geography* work – going from his head, down his body, ending at his toes – beginning in the seventh session. I then constructed an intervention programme, as shown in Table 5, which served as a guide for activities and exercises during the autumn term. However, I felt quite free to select which exercises to do, or not to do, in any particular session, taking my cue from James himself.

Exercise	Aim
1. Hands-on body geography, starting from his head and working downwards – via neck, shoulders, arms, hands, fingers, upper body, waist, legs, feet, toes – accompanied by the naming of respective body parts. Vigorous clapping with his hands, and sometimes his feet.	To foster James' own body awareness and body image. And to strengthen his inner soul experiences of security, trust and confidence.
2. Tactile stimulation by brushing him (literally) on exposed skin areas, and also touching him with contrasting surfaces and objects, e.g. rough or smooth stones, prickly conker case, feather, smooth cold spoon, etc. Also encouraging him to touch/feel these contrasting surfaces.	To help awaken his perceptions for differentiated touch stimuli, and thus exercise his own sense of touch. Also to make him aware, through touch, of his own body boundaries.
3. Walking on my feet, performed by James standing on my feet either with his back towards me or facing me, and with me supporting him.	To enable him to *creep* into my lower senses and, in this way, gain support for his own body senses.
4. Carrying heavy shopping bags as a resistance exercise. Usually with him using two hands to lift one bag, and bringing this to me at the far end of the movement hall. This was sometimes done as a turn-taking exercise.	To come into a stronger experience of gravity and weight, and therefore of his own body.

5. Holding his arms to perform large movements. This could be done while I stood behind James or facing him. Such movements could be circular, vertical or horizontal in/out, contraction/expansion gestures.	To encourage him to relax into making co-ordinated, flowing and/or expansive and contracting arm movements. I felt this has special importance in freeing up his middle or rhythmical system, connected to breathing and speaking. Also to exercise his sense of movement in his own upper limbs.
6. Gross motor activities included: balancing on benches, jumping down from a chair, bouncing on the trampoline, walking, running, etc.	To exercise his lower senses of balance, movement and touch, as the basis for increasing his own body experience and self-awareness.
7. Turn-taking activities, such as receiving/giving a copper rod or a heavy medecine ball, or catching/throwing a lighter ball.	To enter into a social give and take situation. Fostering contact and communication via the objects used.

Table 5. Intervention exercises with James, first half of autumn term, 1998.

SESSION 5: 14 SEPTEMBER, 1998

James came in quietly and I sat him down to put on his eurythmy shoes, similar to plimsolls. He had in fact started to take off his trainers and was perfectly co-operative in letting me put his eurythmy shoes on.

As James was quiet and peaceful I decided to begin with touch activities. I touched him with contrasting objects and surfaces – on his hands (back of hand and palms), cheeks, also his bare feet and lower legs (his shoes/socks were removed for this). He allowed this to be done. Items used included: brushes, plastic/nylon abrasive pad, stones rough/smooth and different shapes, sandpaper, prickly conker case.

Other activities were:

1. *James walking on my feet, with him wearing eurythmy shoes and me normal shoes. His back was towards me, with me holding him with my arms. He appears to recall doing this from last autumn 1997, as he readily puts himself in position for this exercise.*

2. *Walking along wide benches. He fiddles with his fingers and clothing whilst doing this – I encourage him not to fiddle like this. He does this exercise well, maintains his balance, doesn't look unsteady or fall off. In fact he did this exercise after I had been turning around with him, which made me feel slightly dizzy, but he then went to step up on to the bench!*

3. *Carrying shopping bags. He did this willingly, picking up either of the two bags (one is lighter than the other) with two hands. He was able to manage the heavier bag, which shows he has quite some strength.*

4. *He held the copper rod with me standing behind him and holding his hands to raise arms up (all the way) and down. He doesn't put his arms right up in a relaxed way.*

5. *Also passed the medicine ball between us whilst sitting opposite, with me saying 'you and me'. Also did this with the copper rod. James was reciprocating with this (not speaking though).*

I did not run around with James in this session. I took my cues from his rather peaceful state (not hyperventilating heavily – he only really begins to do this when he fiddles rapidly with his clothing).

I was very pleased with this session with James. He was not at all whingy, but surprisingly calm and peaceful. There was no protesting at all. He made some eye contact with me.

SESSION 15: 5 OCTOBER, 1998

I observed James in the playground – he was hopping up and down as he typically does. (It's a sort of skipping he does, up on his toes.) I called his name, he turned, saw me and came.

I went with him to the movement hall. James sat on the chair (where he is now) waiting patiently. He took the initiative to take his shoes off.

Body geography and hand-clapping. He obviously enjoyed this; smiling, twinkling eyes. Now also making contact – putting his face up to me. Did the exercise again. When I physically exert more pressure he finds it amusing, laughs and enjoys it.

Brushing him. By his attentiveness he seems to be registering impressions. Sometimes smiles. Cold spoon on forehead and neck. He came and sat on me.

Walking on my feet. He comes readily for this, his back to me first, then facing me. Stays on my feet very well.

Moving arms up/down, out/in.

In this session James was co-operative, attentive, mainly peaceful.

SESSION 20: 13 OCTOBER, 1998

James was in his usual playtime position today – up on the climbing platform.

When it was 11am I went across and called his name. He responded by looking in my direction. He sat on the slide (which was wet!) and came down that way. Then as we walked away, he turned to me and put his arms around me. Now he sits waiting as usual ready to start.

Body geography, clapping, rubbing hands and feet. James is not very animated today. Not even the clapping brought a smile. According to his teacher, he has quite a cold. But he's co-operative. I started to do the exercise again, combing his hair with my fingers. But he took my hands down and came and sat on me. I gave him some hugs, which he didn't object to.

I tried the exercise again – down his body, starting at the head. But he didn't want this. Sat on me again.

I worked on his feet, rubbing them with rough/smooth surfaces. (He does have quite a runny nose.)

Walked benches, also a narrow one with me supporting him.

Walked a little on my feet.

Then I got the trampoline out. He bounced on this a lot, became more animated and was obviously enjoying it. Makes eye contact. I also gave him some hugs in between bouncing.

Today, as James was possibly not feeling too bright with his cold, I was flexible in what we did.

Results of the intervention process

Looking back at my notes, what changes/results could I identify over this six to seven week period?

- Considerable decrease in hyperventilating.
- More calm and peaceful.
- Reduction in obsessive activity, such as twisting/ fiddling with his clothing.
- Increased eye contact.
- Increased smiling at me.
- Increased co-operation and attentiveness.
- Increased expression of enjoyment and pleasure, e.g. through laughter and liveliness.
- Sometimes taking initiative, e.g. taking his shoes off, coming to sit on me, putting himself into position for walking on my feet.
- Generally less evasive.
- Responding when I call his name, e.g. by looking at me, or coming.

Since a therapeutic process is a two-way involvement, had I noticed any changes in myself over this period? To begin with, I had taken a firm and clear attitude with James, and had wanted him to follow my instructions. I had experienced that this seemed to work well, in that James responded positively and became more settled and secure, as I had provided him with a clear level of expectation. However, as the sessions continued I felt I could be more flexible, sensitive and open towards James and his wishes; partly depending on his state of physical health. A warm and light, humorous or playful approach, with some teasing from me, worked well.

Discussion and evaluation

All the intervention exercises done with James called upon his four lower senses of touch, balance, movement and life. The experiences afforded by the inner sense of life, such as a feeling of well-being, were stimulated by the regular rhythmic occurrence of the sessions, four times a week, at the same time.

The exercises were aimed especially at strengthening James' own body experience through helping his ego to engage, via the lower senses. However, this would in turn help to stimulate his higher (social) senses of word, thought and ego.

For example, it was observed that during touch exercises James would often become very attentive and peaceful and make eye contact with me. As we know, the sense of touch has a particular developmental relationship with the sense of ego (for the recognition of the other person).

It was clear that James responded well to direct physical forms of contact, such as hugs and squeezes, and that he then *warmed up* in terms of his interaction with me – nonverbal communication, eye contact, smiling and expressions of his own enjoyment and pleasure.

The marked decrease in his characteristic hyperventilation during the sessions, his becoming calm and peaceful while sitting on a chair facing me to experience touching, and the decrease in obsessional activities (e.g. fiddling/twisting his clothing), were particularly impressive signs of progress towards better ego-integration.

I therefore had good reason to feel pleased with the way the therapeutic process was going so far.

The perceptions of others

Had other educators, such as James' class teacher or his house-mother at the school, noticed any changes with James over this first period of interventions?

James' house-mother wrote:

James' obsession with tractors/cars has been very strong as well as a new interest in the toilet. He will now go into the toilet by himself but, as yet, will not perform.

He has been more reactive if he is thwarted from play, and makes a fuss when getting ready for bed or if he cannot eat the second he hears the dinner gong.

Physically, James had apparently never been so well as in this first half of the term. James' class teacher wrote:

James' way of walking changed. Rather than bouncing along he now drags his feet, hardly lifting them at all.

He is extremely stubborn, and cries easily if he doesn't get his way.

On the other hand, he is much quieter in the classroom situation and very patient with activities that require sitting behind a desk and sitting still.

After the two-week autumn half-term, James' mother wrote:

James has changed considerably since he has been at your school. He is generally more calm and does not make so many noises (that's good!). He is definitely more aware of his body and I actually feel as if he realises that his legs and feet are attached to his body.

He is also (when at home) continually changing his clothes – this is good in one sense as I feel he is more aware of his body and himself, but he is obsessed with stripy tops.

He has become very stubborn about things and tries to dictate what he wants to wear each day, but with this comes James' ability to choose for himself. He seems less obsessive about his dad's van and not so keen to leg it all the time!

His mother also noticed a clear increase in James' interaction with her in terms of communicating his wishes, and a marked increase in showing interest in his surroundings. James' sister (seventeen months older than James) noticed a clear increase in his communication with other children.

His father had seen some small increases in James' contact and communication with him, but nothing very substantial.

Conclusion

A number of important observations, which provide confirmation of my own work in trying to strengthen James' own body experience and ego-integration, are clearly seen in the above accounts. Namely, that he appeared to be more aware of his body as a connected whole, and also that his way of walking had changed so that he seemed to be more 'grounded'.

On the other hand, he seemed to be more wilful, stubborn and reactive if he could not get his own way. Positively, this could be viewed as stronger self-assertion, in keeping with his actual age (nine years old). The work on his lower senses was intended to increase his bodily awareness as a necessary basis for a stronger inner experience of self.

Both at school and at home James displayed marked obsessional behaviours, and yet, he had also become calmer and quieter, more patient and able to wait in some situations.

Overall, I had the impression that the changes with James were indicative of progress in his own self-awareness, as well as his surroundings, including, at least at home, some communication with other children.

Second half of the autumn term, 1998

In the fifteen sessions following half-term, we continued some of the exercises we had already been practising and stopped others, such as the body geography and tactile stimulation with brushing and objects. Towards the end of term, I introduced some new activities, accompanied by speaking or singing, following an internal review meeting.

Examples taken from the detailed notes of the sessions are given below.

SESSION 29: 17 NOVEMBER, 1998

I started to rub his feet as usual, but James got up and went to the trampoline (which was standing on its side). So I obliged him and put the trampoline down.

James used it vigorously, obviously enjoying it – laughing. In between his using the trampoline, I gave him big squeezes and hugs, which he also enjoyed.

Now he sits quietly again, and I catch his eye! Worked at his feet, and sometimes he looks towards me briefly. Then back to the trampoline; he really enjoys it. More hugs and squeezes.

Now sitting quietly again – entirely peaceful. Then the trampoline again. Plenty of exercise helps contact, emotional responsiveness and interaction. Now sitting again ready to have his socks and shoes put on.

Then carrying the shopping bag. He did it – I praised him – he responded, looked pleased, smiled.

Then arm movements with me standing behind him. He's still too tense; I want to work on this.

I would say a good, responsive session with James – a lot of interaction. He gives back, through his enjoyment in movement, smiles, laughter and eye contact.

SESSION 33: 1 DECEMBER, 1998

I was in the playground and James came to me, so I went to the movement hall with him. He took off his hat, scarf and coat (I unzipped it).

Went into the hall – took his shoes and socks off.

James wanted the trampoline, so we did this first. He enjoys it very much – really laughs.

Now sitting down for a rest; feet up (to be rubbed). Hyperventilating again; he hasn't done this for a long time.

Used the trampoline, then hugs and spins, all of which he enjoys.

He's wilful when he wants his way. His cold is a bit better, no longer has a runny nose. Now he is sitting peacefully.

I let James have his way a good deal, but not always – it's a two-way affair.

A good deal of eye contact and smiling during gross movement activities. He carried the heavy shopping bag, twice.

Finally I tried to move his arms in small upward curves (similar to the movements for the 'L' sound in eurythmy). This is not easy as he readily stiffens and resists. However I plan to improve on this.

Session 38: 15 December, 1998

First foot rubbing. He wanted the trampoline straight away, but I made it clear he'd have to wait, which he did.

Then trampoline, hugs, spins. Now sitting on chair waiting. Did the anapest rhythm (short, short, long) to the verse 'Brave and true I will be'. Clapping it with me holding his hands, and then stamping it by me holding his lower legs/ankles. I sat James on the low bench, rather than the chair, so that I could really stamp his feet on the floor. We did this rhythm several times.

Then, 'Row, row, row your boat gently down the stream', while sitting down and holding the copper rod between us. James held the rod and went with the movement.

Then ball passing while sitting down and while standing. He has no clear notion, or skill, how to catch and throw a ball. I feel this should be learnt.

Then moving his arms, with me taking his wrists/hands and making the movements – in and out, up and round. He went with it; very well actually, didn't stiffen up or resist.

Results of the intervention process

It would be true to say that the behaviours and responses listed before half-term were maintained in the second half of term, but without any obvious changes in their levels of attainment. The one exception was an increased expression of enjoyment and pleasure by James, due to changed exercises – more extensive use of the trampoline and frequent physical hands-on contact. With the latter, the rougher the better as far as he was concerned! As I noted after Session 25:

> James actually shows a good deal of emotional and contact/communication responsiveness when in a situation that he enjoys. I find this to be a real emotional (affective) feedback, such as one would not expect to find in a deeply autistic child. He also responds to teasing and playfulness.

Considering that James had a cold for much of the second half of term (he is prone to colds and catarrh) he still maintained an impressive level of participation and responsiveness. In Session 31, for example, he continued to thoroughly enjoy using the trampoline and receiving bear hugs, despite having both a cold and cough.

My notes contained only occasional mention of any obsessional behaviours during the sessions, and this was similar with his hyper-ventilating.

Discussion and evaluation

As far as I was concerned – and I believe James felt likewise – the sessions had gone well, with a good deal of interaction between us.

The exercises had again strongly called upon the functioning of his lower (body) senses, and the overall aim of increasing his own body awareness and self-experience, and thereby of fostering his personal and social awareness. However, it was interesting to note how James tended to alternate between looking rather deadpan, often while sitting on a chair, and becoming very animated, lively and cheerful during very physical activities.

Unfortunately there were no signs of any speech development, with no clear syllables or sounds.

The perceptions of others

An internal review meeting took place at the school on 7 December after 34 sessions with James. What follows is derived, firstly, from the record of this review, and then his parents' observations during the three-week Christmas holiday.

His house-mother reported changes since the autumn half-term:

> James' obsessive behaviours became more intense, and there were also more of them. For example, obsessed with getting the cutlery containers, he will get out of bed in the morning to find these. Obsession with stripy jumpers, which he wants on and off. In these behaviours he hyperventilates and has a manic impression.
>
> When the first gong goes in the house (to signal ten minutes to lunchtime), James immediately wants food. Sometimes he laughs, occasionally tears. You often don't know why he reacts as he does.
>
> Since half-term there have been five occasions of soiling and poking himself (though not masturbation). The fifth incident was a major event, with faeces around the dormitory. Previously James has never liked to be dirty, but this has now changed to an oblivion of being dirty!
>
> James has become more aware of sensory matters relating to his own body – he is into his lower senses. A couple of days ago, and for the first time, James wanted grown-ups to tickle his knees!

In the review meeting the medical adviser asked if there had been any changes in James' environment at school since half-term. The house-mother explained that a new pupil came, who now shares a room with James. He started as a day pupil, and then as a weekly boarder. However, she did not feel that this had influenced James particularly.

Had any improvements been seen with James since half-term? The house-mother's answer was a clear *no*.

James' class teacher reported that:

> He had shown strong obsessive behaviour in the class
> since half-term, expressed by him going for music stands
> at the slightest opportunity.

How then did James appear to his parents during the holidays? His
mother wrote that:

> James is really getting to know what he does/does not
> want to do, but because he is unable to express himself
> verbally he gets very frustrated. He appears to have a
> greater understanding of himself. He is more aware of his
> body and his feelings. This, however, means he is not so
> easy to persuade, and if he has made his mind up about
> something, that's it! I think that in the long term this is all
> good. It's just a question of enabling him to communicate
> without shrieking and being so stubborn.

His mother had also observed a marked increase in James engaging
in two-way communication with her but, interestingly, a decrease in
communicating his own wishes.

His father had noticed slight decreases in James' contact and
communication with him.

Conclusion

Whereas I continued to have very positive experiences with James in
our sessions together, others were reporting new changes of a difficult
and problematic nature for them – if not for James himself! The
medical adviser was able to throw a very helpful light on this, from an
anthroposophic perspective.

Bearing in mind that the clear aim of the interventions was
to facilitate James' ego-integration – the penetration of his soul-
spiritual nature into his physical life body – we could interpret the

problematic changes and developments as a part of this deeper incarnation process.

The stronger obsessive behaviours, the greed for food, the increased self-will, were expressive of James' astrality (the astral body carries soul wishes and desires). It appeared therefore that he was now becoming more involved with his soul-astral nature. Together with this was a growing awareness of, and penetration into, his actual physical body. This was evident from James walking more on the ground and less on tiptoe, an awareness of his limbs, and perhaps even his interest in poking himself and soiling, which had never been known before.

What was then required to aid this incarnation process further, beyond just the astral nature? It would need therapeutic exercises to engage James' ego (the spirit), so that the ego could help to bring order, peace and direction into the rather wild astral nature from which the obsessions arose.

The medical adviser recommended exercises combining speech with rhythm and movement. Interestingly, in all the work I had done with James before the review meeting, I had not consciously incorporated speech. After the review I immediately took up this recommendation. Furthermore, the doctor said that he could understand (and would even have expected) that by stimulating an incarnation process in James, his behaviour could 'get worse before it became better'. Both resistance and aggravation from the child can become evident as soon as you encourage 'a more incarnated situation'.

It was agreed that I should continue with my sessions during the spring term after the three-week Christmas holiday, but three times a week rather than four.

Spring term, 1999

During the twenty sessions until the end of March, there were some changes to the exercises, as well as continuity from the end of the previous term. In particular, I decided to stop using the trampoline, because I did not want this to be the main focus of James' attention at the expense of other helpful activities.

Session 3: 20 January, 1999

James came willingly with me into the movement hall. We sat down and he put his feet up for his socks to be taken off. I worked on his feet. (His hands were warm today, his feet coldish.) He did some hyperventilating.

Then we did the anapest rhythm (short, short, long) accompanied by speech, 'Brave and true I will be'; first clapping then stamping. He seems to enjoy it; smiling and looking at me. The more vigorously done, the better.

Now he's gone off bench walking again. (James had taken the initiative to walk along the benches, at the sides of the movement hall, since the first session this term.)

Hugs and spins. Obviously enjoyed it. Very direct eye contact.

Then did the other rhythmic exercise, 'Row, row, row your boat'. He was smiling throughout.

Hyperventilating stopped – very calm as I rubbed his feet.

Big arm movements – he went with this – up and round, in and out. Stiffened once. But then when I had to put his boots on to take him back to class, big protest. Definitely didn't want this (the boots I think).

However, had to be!

Session 7: 2 February, 1999

At break time James was making a big fuss. Apparently he wanted to get into the classroom to the music stand.

I've rubbed his feet – he sat peacefully for that – apart from breathing a bit noisily.

Now he's walking along the benches. We've had eye contact and smiling. (He's still got a cold, but not coughing.) Hands warm, feet cool.

Now he's touching the wall – fingers in the gaps between the blocks – interested in the wall?

Hugs, spins. He liked this, smiled and laughed.

Game – 'You can't catch me' – really interrelating.

Sat down again – peaceful.

Did the 'Brave and true' rhythm. He often gives the impression of enjoying this. Then 'Row, row, row your boat'. He holds the copper rod, looks at me directly, smiling. (I do feel I have good, positive, contact with James.)

Now bench walking again in between. I still want to do arm movements – ball/rod throwing/passing to get his arms and hands in use.

I experienced this as a good session, with interaction, contact and communication. James co-operated. No protests.

Session 20: 30 March, 1999 (the last one this term)

James came with me before the bell went. I find him more with it in the impression he gives, and the way he looks at me.

Foot rubbing first.

Did the rhythm with speech – he resisted going with me at times.

Then hugs/spins/chasing.

Then rowing with singing – peaceful – eye contact is good when it takes place. I do feel I can meet James in this eye contact.

Now he's taken off his jumper and is standing on a bench. Breathing through his mouth. He still has quite a cold.

At times James was protesting a bit today. Co-operated mainly, but at times screeching/whining a bit. He does this, I presume, to say that he doesn't want any more – that it's enough!

Did some large arm movements with him – up and round, in and out. Could do some, but he stiffens up when he doesn't want to do them.

At the end he went quite happily with me back to the classroom.

Results of the intervention process

Usually the sessions went well, with a good deal of contact and communication taking place.

- ⁂ More direct eye contact in which I felt we really met.
- ⁂ The impression that James was often more with it; more there and open, less distant and aloof.
- ⁂ He was more interactive, e.g. in playing a chasing game, or in responding to teasing.

- ❋ Sometimes resisted in an exercise, so it had to be achieved with his willing co-operation.
- ❋ Generally he warmed up during a session, and there was more contact, interaction and involvement as we proceeded.
- ❋ He took the initiative to go bench walking and touching the walls of the hall, rather like marking out the boundaries.
- ❋ Interestingly, while I felt thoroughly dizzy after spinning, he showed little, if any, signs of dizziness.
- ❋ Although he continued to have colds and often a runny nose, mostly this did not appear to hamper him from becoming active and enjoying himself.
- ❋ Sometimes he would be more relaxed in making arm movements with me, but often he would stiffen up. This was an activity he couldn't readily enter into.
- ❋ He generally participated well in the rhythmic exercises, which also involved arm movements, such as clapping and rowing.
- ❋ He was not yet able to catch or throw a ball or a rod.
- ❋ I was not aware of any obsessional behaviours in the sessions.

Discussion and evaluation

The warming-up phenomenon of James becoming more animated, alive and participating as we got into a session is, I think, very important. Even in physical terms I could see the difference in James' responsiveness if he was warmly dressed. On the soul level, a warm, light-hearted, friendly approach from me met with a positive response from him, which showed James' ability to reciprocate appropriately.

From anthroposophy we know that warmth is the element that provides the link between the physical and the spiritual levels. The human ego (spirit) lives in the warmth and, within the body, warm blood is the vehicle or bearer of the ego.

Therefore warmth on the physical, soul and spiritual levels was very important to help James' process of ego-integration and his human, social interaction. He could also then respond to me in a warm, friendly way.

It was also important to ask the question, 'When is James more present or more distant?' and to be sensitive in order to perceive these situations. Clearly in physical contact activities he was there, making eye contact and smiling, but he was also more present when he was peaceful and calm. The 'Row your boat' exercise had a calming effect, and could be accompanied by good eye contact and smiling.

However, the lack of any obvious dizziness on his part (not mine!) after whole body spins performed by me holding him from behind, under his arms and around his chest, did perhaps suggest a lack of being centred in himself.

Bench walking and touching the wall of his own initiative might be seen as exploring the boundaries of the room, as he was also becoming more aware of the boundaries of his own physical body.

His difficulty to relax sufficiently when making large arm movements with me in the vertical and horizontal planes, as well as an inability to catch and throw a ball, seemed to reflect a tightness or lack of freedom in his middle, rhythmical system. There was also no indication of any development, however slight, towards speech. I also noticed no clear imitative ability with James in the realm of movements.

However, overall, I felt that progress had been made in engaging James, and making more direct, interpersonal contact with him.

The perceptions of others

The internal review meeting took place on 29 March, 1999, the day before my last intervention session with James.

His house-mother reported that:

> Leading up to Christmas, James had presented the picture
> of a rather unhappy and disturbed boy. However, when he

returned to school for the start of the spring term, James was in a far better state.

He was much calmer and more in control, and less obsessive. He was more responsive now to challenges, but also showed greater resistance and self-assertiveness. More self-willed.

In the realm of communication he seemed to be at a standstill, and the important question raised was how to help James make further steps in the area of language and communication. Seemingly, in the daily pattern of life, James understood basics.

A totally new development was that he was now willing to take medicines, whereas previously this had been a constant battle!

The class teacher confirmed that:

James was much calmer now, more balanced, without the mood swings he had shown last term.

His strong obsession with music stands had completely fallen away, and he now showed no interest in them.

He was more open to doing things now, and it was much easier for him to sit and wait. He was more relaxed in class.

There was an issue of him wanting to be in charge.

James liked games and activities that involved turn-taking.

Importantly, in both house and class, there were small signs that James was taking more interest in other children.

I received a letter from James' mother towards the end of April, to share his parents' perceptions during the Easter holidays.

Dear Bob
Re: James
Thank you very much for your letter. Before we received the letter we had noticed how much more openly and

spontaneously affectionate he has been. This has also been noticed by other people who are close to James. He cuddles without asking, comes into bed in the morning and just generally seems to want attention and to be around people. Although, on occasion, James had done these things in the past, it has usually taken a great deal of effort on his part and indeed ours!

The improvement in James since you have been working with him is incredible. I think I fed back to you in the beginning how he now realises his feet are attached to his body and he actually owns them! It gave me great pleasure the other day when we were out walking that he kept lifting up his foot for me to tie his shoelaces.

James still has his obsessions and at the moment it is jumpers with zips and his dad's van, but what is great about that is that he can actually do up zips.

We would like to thank you again for all the time you spend working with and helping James; it really is appreciated and quite obviously paying dividends.

Conclusion

It seemed clear that the crisis of the second half of the autumn term had been surmounted, and that James had progressed to a new level of balance within himself and in relation to his surroundings. He was both calmer and more self-assertive, and importantly, more in control of himself.

This suggested that steps were being achieved in the process of ego-integration, which included overcoming James' obsessions arising from his undirected astrality. He appeared to be more in charge of his life, and to be able to express his affections for others.

As our medical adviser had said in the December review meeting, things 'may get worse before they get better'. This appeared to have been very clearly borne out by the latest reports and observations.

It seems reasonable to conclude that the intensive, one-to-one interventional process had made a significant impact on James' positive overall progress – that is, in alleviating his former degree of autistic withdrawal and aloofness, and in fostering greater participation, interest and involvement with others. No other special therapies or treatments had taken place during the intervention period. Therefore, the evidence presented does, I believe, strongly support the value and effectiveness of the interventional process with James.

It is, however, important to note that in the course of such a planned process, a child may go through a period of greater difficulties, such as more intense obsessional behaviour, which can be interpreted as a result of the deeper processes of incarnation and ego-integration which were taking place (see Chapters 3 and 4).

Confirmations of progress

The interventions stopped at the end of March, and in the annual review meeting in June and the annual school and house reports in July, the following significant remarks were recorded.

James' mother:

> ...is very pleased with James' growing involvement to be in a group. She and James' family have noticed that James is more mature, calmer and more observant. During a conversation James looks from one person to the other ... His obsessions are still strong at home. She has been encouraging James to be more upright when walking and to lift his head up and make more eye contact. She has observed a lot more involvement with other children.

James' house-mother at school:

> James has progressed well with self-help skills and begins to take a little initiative. He has gained more confidence and one can demand more from him to do things with

a greater independence. Recently there has been direct contact with other children, and James has shown an interest and warmth towards them, which so far had not occurred.

James' class teacher:

> James is in a class with seven other children. He is well liked by the others and even though he is still more adult-orientated he does show more and more interest in his peers. He does not seem to be so much of a loner any more but is always right in the centre with all the other children.

When James returned to school in September 1999 after the long summer holidays, an important new change had occurred. He was toilet-trained and now took himself to the toilet whenever he needed it! This breakthrough, age ten, was further clear evidence of a new bodily awareness and inner self-experience that had developed in James following our intervention sessions.

A final word

In this chapter we have seen how the anthroposophic model of autism has been practically implemented within the broad context of curative education. This holistic model generates specific therapeutic attitudes and intervention exercises, which can help to alleviate the degree of autism shown by individual children. The educator's awareness and recognition of the child's unique spiritual being is a crucial factor in the attempt to build empathetic and supportive interrelationships with each child, and clearly encourages increased mutual contact and communication.

As is the case with most of us, we respond positively and become more open and relaxed when we sense and feel that we are both understood and recognised in our uniqueness by others.

155

8. Autism and the Senses

MARI STERTEN

The work of Woodward and authors cited in this book are highly relevant today. Over recent years more awareness and attention has been given to the possible effects of the varying functioning of the senses in people diagnosed with ASD (autism spectrum disorder).

A number of accounts by people diagnosed with ASD have come into the public eye, which, not least, are calling attention to the sensory difficulties common in autism. Donna Williams, famous for books and lecture tours on her condition, says:

> For me, sensory hypersensitivity is a fluctuating condition which rests on information overload. It can be a chronic problem due to the chronic problem of overload. Information overload is due to problems of connection. When hearing becomes acute, it is because too much information is coming in for the brain to keep up with its connections, then the perception of these sounds becomes intensely unbearable. The same thing can happen with touch. When I have taken in a lot of visual or sound information, my sense of touch can be overly sensitive, sharp as a pin, to be touched can be as shocking as to be jolted. (Williams 1998, 202)

And Temple Grandin says:

> Sudden loud noises hurt my ears like a dentist's drill hitting a nerve ... An autistic child will cover his or her

ears because certain sounds hurt; it is like an excessive
startle reaction. High-pitched shrill noises are the worst.
But common noises like school bells, the scraping
of chairs or the squeaking of microphones can cause
discomfort, and anticipation of painful noise can trigger
difficult behaviours hours in advance. (Grandin 2000)

Tito Mukhopadhyay says that people with autism, at least those
who are like him, choose one sensory channel. He chose hearing.
Most of the time, Tito attends to the sounds of language and to oral
information, which may help explain his gift for poetry. Vision, Tito
said, is painful. He scans the world with his peripheral vision and rarely
looks directly at anything (Blakeslee 2002).

These and other accounts have led to greater insights into the
irregular sense perceptions often experienced by people with autism,
and the drastic impact these can have on well-being, state of tension
and ability to communicate, or functioning in general.

Work pioneered by behaviourist Rimland (1964); Delacato (1974),
who developed the Delacato method of neurological rehabilitation in
autism using sensory therapy; the Sensory Integration research work
of A. Jane Ayres (1989), an occupational therapist who developed
S. I. theory and practice in the 1960s, which is now widely used in
occupational therapy; and the sensory modulation and motor output
in autism research by Ornitz (1989) find echoes and are developed
further in today's neuropsychology and neuroscience. Eminent neu-
roscientist Michael Merzenich is a leading authority in the field of
neuroplasticity. He has made strong contributions to the field of rehabilitation and recovery after brain trauma, and his work also includes
training programmes specifically directed to brain development and
learning in autism, which have proved effective for part of the autistic
population.

It has been noted by some researchers that the brains
of autistic children are larger than average and that the
brain's basic building blocks, called cortical columns,

contain many more cells than normal and make excess
connections to other cells. Such hyper-connectivity
may cause autistic children to become overwhelmed by
details because their minds are never free to integrate the
whole picture. Moreover, their brains are wired in such
a way that they are prone to associate things that do not
normally go together. (Blakeslee 2002)

In a marked difference to old-fashioned behavioural therapy born
out of a 'determined from the outside' tabula rasa view of the human
being, today the accent is much more one of acceptance of and respect
for each individual; and on nurturing human relationships that place
the child or vulnerable person in the centre of an interactive environment, adaptive to the needs of the individual, where mutual development and learning takes place. This model is well known from curative
education and the 'ecological framework' of social pedagogy.

The person-centred approach places great store on empathy and
genuine acceptance, which indeed can lead to deeper levels of recognition. Phoebe Caldwell's brand of 'intensive interaction' (originally
coined and developed by Dave Hewett's team in 1989/90) is an inspi-
rational method of reaching children on the autistic spectrum, forming
relationships and communicating using 'their language': individual
body language. The simple lyrics from well-known band The Who's
album, *Tommy* – 'See me, feel me, touch me, heal me' – embody the
need for the fundamental basis of human development: to interact and
form relationships with the world, and *become*. Modern catchwords
like 'empowerment' and 'autonomy' reflect a gradual change in attitude
over the last twenty years, with greater sensitivity to the individual's
situation and needs. When these needs are recognised and mutually
met, empathetic responses can lead to better thriving, health and resilience, a better quality of life, improved possibilities for learning and an
improved prognosis for the future. In a culture with good and healthy
rhythms of life and positive relationships, the nervous system and
organic functions can be positively affected and may to some extent be
able to 'repair' themselves.

Understanding and responding

A number of nervous-system based difficulties are associated with autism, including sensory and information processing problems. In her book *Sensory Perceptual Issues in Autism and Asperger Syndrome*, researcher and mother Olga Bogdashina (2003) writes about a number of possible sensory experiences in autism: literal perception, the inability to filter out information (executive functioning), hypersensitivity and/ or hyposensitivity, inconsistency of sensory perception, fragmented perception, distorted perception, sensory agnosia, delayed processing and vulnerability to overload. Different perceptual styles seen in autism can include mono-processing, peripheral perception and sensory compensation. Mono-processing entails being able to consciously use only one main sensory channel, such sight, and whilst taking note of every visual detail, all other information vanishes into the background. Peripheral perception is the phenomenon of avoiding direct perception (such as direct eye contact, focused visual perception and focused tactile perception) because it is too 'strong', it 'hurts'; the experience is too overwhelming. To compensate for visual distortions and meaning-blindness, tapping, smelling or licking (among other examples) may be used to aid the processing of incoming information about the environment. Eyes and ears function, but distortions may be experienced, and processing through vision and hearing alone is not enough.

> If there is too much in the way of floating and
> unprocessed images, sounds and sensations, the brain
> may interpret this sensory information as threatening, to
> the point where it triggers the body's self defence system
> ... children retreat into repetitive behaviours, isolating
> themselves from disturbing input. Here they can at least
> focus on something that makes sense ... Rather than
> understanding that the child is experiencing extreme
> painful sensory overload ... those of us who are not on the
> autistic spectrum see the child's behaviour as it affects us;
> the child is having a tantrum. (Caldwell 2010)

Furthermore there are known issues of attention and memory as they may manifest in autism, and these again affect concept formation. (Bogdashina 2003, 44)

It is clearly important to observe and attempt to identify all difficulties in order to find therapeutic or remedial responses and approaches when supporting people with ASD. As functioning in autism depends on diverse factors, and well-being and the lowering of stress levels are of primary importance, it is essential to take sensory issues and their impact on functioning into account. Many of the young people I work with do not express themselves through spoken language, so recognising their problems needs careful observation and analysis.

A regularly reviewed sensory profile (Bogdashina's profile is available in her book, 2003) can be a useful tool for becoming more aware of the situation the young person has to manage. It can prove a helpful part of an overall assessment, which should result in an adapted approach and environment that promotes the best possible learning and functioning, including a good temporal life structure.

The 'lower' or bodily senses

Tito Mukhopadhyay wrote, while living in India:

> When I was four or five years old I hardly realised that I had
> a body except when I was hungry or when I realised that
> I was standing under the shower and my body got wet. I
> needed constant movement, which made me get the feeling
> of my body. The movement can be of a rotating type or
> just flapping of my hands. Every movement is a proof that I
> exist. I exist because I can move (Blakeslee 2002).

Dr Marga Hogenboom asked me to contribute a chapter to this book because aspects of my work and the therapeutic exercises I use with children and young people affected by ASD here in Camphill

School Aberdeen have some similarity to the work Bob Woodward describes in this book. My work has evolved out of curative education; in addition I include elements from intensive interaction, Sensory Integration, eurythmy and neurodevelopmental movement, and the remedial work known as 'The Extra Lesson' by Audrey McAllen. It strongly addresses what in anthroposophic sense physiology is termed the 'lower senses', which all relate to being grounded and in our bodily self. The four lower senses give us the fundament of bodily identity:

> Tito, who is fourteen, often stops the testing with bursts
> of activity. His body rocks rhythmically. He stands and
> spins. He makes loud smacking noises. Everyone waits.
> Tito reaches for a yellow pad and writes to explain
> his behaviour, 'I am calming myself. My senses are so
> disconnected, I lose my body. So I flap. If I don't do this, I
> feel scattered and anxious'. (Blakeslee 2002)

One way of addressing these and similar difficulties is by means of Sensory Integration therapy, which aims to balance arousal levels in order to maximise attention span and the ability to engage 'presence'. It uses activities primarily directed at integrating the lower senses: sense of touch, sense of balance (informing body posture and righting reflexes) and sense of proprioception or movement (muscles and joints, giving information about the body in space). Using physical lower sense experiences to focus attention can enhance the co-ordination of vision, rhythm/timing, movement and also speech, and lead to enhanced general ability.

With my work I attempt to address well-being through movement and rhythm, stimulating blood circulation, healthy organic processes, relaxed breathing and, where possible, the experience of fluid movement co-ordination.

The basis of therapy is a respectful and empathetic relationship. On a soul level, I attempt to promote trust, the experience of competence, confidence and as a by-product, resilience.

The term *kinaesthetic* corresponds to the *sense of movement* in anthroposophic terminology. *Proprioception* (own perception) is also strongly related to the sense of movement: the sense of the relative position of neighbouring parts of the body and strength of effort being employed in movement. It is distinguished from *interoception* (or the *sense of life* in anthroposophic terms), which senses the physiological condition of the entire body and the ability of visceral information to reach awareness and affect behaviour, directly or indirectly; for example, informing our inner state of hunger, pain and well-being, which are strongly influenced by the reactions of the autonomous nervous system. The sense of *equilibrium*, situated in the inner ear, informs our postural system and helps us maintain head orientation and uprightness. The *tactile* sense or sense of *touch* informs our discrimination in the physical sensory environment and of our own body, including boundaries. All these contribute to a *filled body identity*.

Readers familiar with authors like the already cited Donna Williams, Temple Grandin and Tito Mukhopadhyay will also be familiar with descriptions of unusual own body perceptions and incomplete body maps. These might seem to be linked to atypically developed nervous systems, not able to modulate and process information. The lower, mostly not so conscious, bodily senses, inform the nervous system of the filled body identity, and the internal body map (body scheme) arises, often disturbed in the atypical nervous system of a person with ASD. The following excerpt is from an article published by the *New York Times*. Tito's experiences and the findings of the researchers further describe difficulties faced by people with ASD.

> Tito seems to lack a sense of his own body, the kind of
> internal map, Dr Merzenich said, that normal children
> develop in their first few years. The maps involve
> brain regions that specialise in the sense of touch and
> movement and are widely connected to other areas, and
> they are highly dynamic throughout life, changing in
> response to everyday experience. By imaging the brains
> of higher functioning autistic people who can stay still
> in scanners, researchers in the laboratory of Dr Eric

Courchesne at the University of California at San Diego
found that autistic people had mixed-up brain maps.

Although a normal person, for example, has a well-
defined brain area that specialises in face recognition,
some autistic people have face-recognition areas in parts
of the brain like the frontal lobes, where no one had
dreamed they could be laid down. The same is true of
maps that help plan movements. This means body maps
are formed in autistic children, but they may be scrambled
differently in each person. (Blakeslee 2002)

Particularly proprioception, experienced when 'working against
gravity', offers a stabilising and grounding experience.

The therapeutic exercises

Components

I can see very clear benefits to the young people I work with, reflected
in increased movement skills, well-being and self-esteem, nourished
through the sessions. My hope is that these shall lead to greater general
ability to engage, greater competence, and to an improved resilience.
The therapeutic work is formed in the following way:

- The therapeutic relationship and environment.
- The build-up of exercises: presence of rhythm, exercise
  of co-ordination and timing, balance, working against
  gravity/resistance, challenges on equipment, fine
  co-ordination/tabletop activities.
- Being challenged at the right level leads to successful
  accomplishment and increased ability and self-esteem.
  Exercising choice, free play important.
- A continuous process of assessment and adaptation

The therapeutic relationship is based on careful observation paired with acceptance, positive support, seeking out the young person's strengths, objective warmth and attempted empathy. What makes someone bang the wall with his or her hand, tap things, squint his or her eyes or constantly hum? How can I, in a friendly, unobtrusive manner, give a message that conveys recognition, and create the basis for some mutual interaction? I find I use elements of Phoebe Caldwell's intensive interaction insights in trying to recognise the soul experience, likes and dislikes of the young person. Intensive interaction uses body language to communicate with children and adults in a way that establishes attention and emotional engagement. Phoebe's approach to senses and communication helps develop observation and awareness of subtleties in the child's responses and behaviours, leading to a deeper understanding of what the child may experience, and to appropriate responses.

The ARC model, briefly outlined below, highlights principles I apply which may be of interest to others working in similar fields.

According to Deci and Ryan (2000, and cited in Ziviani *et al.* 2013), the ARC model of the three basic psychological needs, when satisfied, leads to well-being and optimal functioning. Here is the threefold ARC model summed up:

Autonomy: I have choices.
Relatedness: I am connected.
Competence: I can do things.

My observation is that the meeting of these needs charges positive motivation, creates a positive cycle, and fuels spiralling development.

Choice primarily involves discrimination, which belongs to the field of thinking; relatedness is directly linked to emotional development and well-being; and competence to the ability to actively apply one's will forces. These are the three fundamental forces in our soul: thinking, feeling and willing. In Steiner-Waldorf education the teachers learn the importance of addressing and strengthening these three in the way they build up and structure their lessons for different age-groups, for optimal engagement, health and learning.

165

Examples of exercises and activities

My sessions tend to start with an 'arriving exercise' from eurythmy or Bothmer gym, then a verse, done with gestures involving gross and finer co-ordination, grading and flow. Speaking and moving the verse might be done alternatively. I also tend to close sessions with a formal movement exercise, e.g. from eurythmy.

With younger children, I use walking in time to a song and tambourine to get a healthy rhythm of breath and pulse, or an increase/decrease speed exercise, for example with giant steps and gnomie steps. This may be followed by various developmental movement exercises involving co-ordination and proprioception, such as variations of creeping, crawling, bringing together the upper and lower extremities. I have various songs and rhymes for animal images to accompany these, and a simple imaginative sequence makes it a story game. For children over the age of eleven, I use more challenging hopping, jumping, one leg, two legs, wide/together or wide/cross, toe/heel sequences, accompanied by poems, rhymes or songs.

Balance, co-ordination (and singing!) can be practised while bouncing on body balls. With older ones, we might have jogging circuits or lemniscates, where going slowly is more difficult than going quickly.

Weight bearing, to strengthen the upper torso and shoulder girdle, can be done by walking on hands playing wheelbarrow, or over a physio roll, depending on strength and skill.

For hand-eye co-ordination, integrating right and left, above and below, various exercises with elements of eurythmy using rods and beanbags are helpful, and singing again enhances the flow.

For proprioception, balance and co-ordination, slow 'deep muscle' strengthening, through balancing and concentrating exercises, some inspired from yoga or pilates, can be very good for increasing movement control and presence.

After finishing their prescribed exercises, the children are free to experiment with equipment. First they have to communicate their choices, using photo cards and speech where possible, then help to hang up their equipment and place mats appropriately. My store of equipment includes, among other things: a large body ball for balance and body feedback (sense of proprioception, touch, vestibular sense); a bolster swing for balance and proprioception; a net swing for postural exercises, proprioception, deep pressure and vestibular stimulation; rings and bar for proprioception and vestibular stimulation; a platform swing for postural exercises and vestibular integration; and a tyre-tube swing. I also have materials for typical tabletop activities: drawing, cutting and pasting, modelling, sewing on card, spoke weaving, basket weaving, felting etc. Sewing and weaving can also be combined, for example, with sitting in the net.

HOPED FOR OUTCOMES

- Body schema experiencing resistance, gravity, proprioception, leading to an improved sense of bodily identity and stability.
- Reducing anxiety, hypersensitivity, improving 'optimal arousal levels', state of inner balance and presence for optimal ability to function.
- Regulating breathing, feeling safe, understanding what goes on – predictability, sequences and routines, visual aids, timetables, trusting relationships.
- Autonomy, choices, empowerment, success, confidence, competence.

Case study: Johnny

A sensitive youngster, poorly built-up physical body and muscular system (possibly effected by neglect), difficult to close mouth, prone to colds, cold extremities, poor blood circulation, asthma. Diagnosis of autism.

Poor language processing, dependent on visual clues and body language; poor and limited speech (aphasia), able to recognise and read many words and in that context can say words quite clearly.

167

Emotionally very insecure, Johnny takes a long time to build up confidence and safety in relationships, relies heavily on routines for orientation and sense of what is expected. He may, when unsettled due to not quite grasping what is happening, act in an ADHD anxious/ aggravated manner.

Johnny can be at the mercy of obsessively repeated actions, particularly to restore any physical object shifted by others to its original place, to keep things the same and be 'in control'.

Johnny struggles to understand and to cope with everyday demands: being present in class, focusing on tasks. He finds changes, especially those of people, hard to handle. Johnny is oversensitive to sound and acutely aware visually. He has a near photographic memory of written words, but struggles with meaning of language. He can be very impatient and restless, and has a low tolerance threshold; his frustration can easily escalate into violence, but also easily de-escalate with the help of people who know him well.

EXERCISE PROGRAMME

Johnny's therapeutic exercise programme has proprioceptive components, to support body awareness, strength and co-ordination. It employs rhythm, neurodevelopmental movement patterns and postural exercises. It also employs eurythmy gestures, speech and fine co-ordination.

Success is a very important component, leading to more competence and, hopefully, transferable well-being and confidence. The expectations are made as clear as possible, the sequence of movements is built up over time, and each achievement is celebrated.

Initially Johnny's motivation was strongly fired by the prospect of getting to swing in the net or on the bolster, causing him to repeatedly ask, 'Push, please.' He had no difficulty showing me which equipment he wanted or the corresponding picture, but had great difficulty remembering the spoken name of the piece of equipment unless it was written on the picture.

As the aim is to increase own function, I would not push him but leave him to propel himself, and after much practice he has achieved the necessary co-ordination of upper and lower body. Getting up onto and balancing on equipment is in itself a challenge, giving lots of body feedback, proprioception and deep pressure whilst placing demands on his postural and balancing abilities.

EXCERPT FROM SESSION NOTES, APRIL 2012, AGED FOURTEEN

Verse with eurythmy gestures: he lets arms drop immediately, does not sustain a raised arm gesture. He finds it difficult to enter into it properly. He does speak some of the words singly, the most familiar beginning and end words.

We hop on one foot holding hands, not so easy although he has buoyancy. He imitates hopping from wide to crossed feet to wide again; we repeat this a number of times. I praise him because he is genuinely making an effort and doing well. We balance on toes, walk on the heels.

My observation is that his movements need penetrating and enlivening; they can be hurried, a bit mechanical and also floppy. The more harmonious and secure he can be in himself, the more he will be able to increase his ability with 'simple' skills, leading to a growth in confidence, a positive cycle! If I can 'catch' his attention he can focus well for spurts of eight to fifteen minutes. It depends on a number of factors, as he is very obsessive. Every little experience of achievement through effort is an important building block towards developing further potential.

EXCERPT FROM AN INTERNAL REPORT (FOR JOHNNY'S PUPIL STUDY), MAY 2012

Arms: We work at penetrating and enlivening the arms with eurythmy gestures; the vowels by themselves and with sounding, and a verse including expansion/contraction. He shows improvement in sustaining attention and performing the actions. He shows lacking sustaining power/vitality, e.g. in raising his arms and holding them up.

Fine footwork: He hops fairly well on one foot, jumps wide/cross/wide, toe walking/heel walking rhythms. These are exercises to help him penetrate his will (also improving his ability to speak).

Sounding/speaking: Part of the session is spent practising closing the mouth and shaping sounds in front of the mirror. He speaks part of the verse and joins sounding for vowels, also other words in conjunction with naming (and occasional self-initiated reading) activities.

Integrating above/below, right/left rhythm: Rod and beanbag exercises, for exercising rhythm/flow, balance and co-ordination.

Developmental creeping/crawling exercises: for co-ordination and proprioception.

Strength: He then gets strengthening exercises, e.g. wheelbarrow walk, work on the ball (weight-bearing/pushing), rings or bar. It can be hard for Johnny to contain himself and make focused efforts when challenged on the equipment, but he is helped by the challenge of the height of the equipment. He loves to get on the swings, and is open to doing more difficult things. He is tasked to learn to sustain presence and grip on the equipment, also to regulate alternating gripping and letting go, using the rope to propel himself – not easy for him.

Motivation/response: Johnny is focused and motivated as long as the challenges are within a successful end range for him. He enjoys feeling that he can do things, can manage. His response is very good.

END OF SCHOOL YEAR REPORT, 2012, AGED FIFTEEN

Johnny has attended weekly with six absences over the year.

Aims: To improve body scheme (perception of own body), balance, co-ordination, attention, and build confidence and strength.

Responses: Johnny co-operates and engages very well. He has made clear progress and improved with postural exercises to strengthen his ability to balance and to co-ordinate arms and legs. Johnny finds it hard to sustain *gestures and movements using his upper extremities, and benefits from exercises aimed to strengthen these and his torso. His timing and flow is improving.*

Johnny always enjoys making use of suspended equipment and work on the large ball. He has a clear sense of achievement, enjoys coming and is well motivated.

Johnny joins in speaking a verse at the beginning of sessions, and is encouraged to name parts of the body, colours, shapes etc.

It would benefit Johnny to continue next school year.

Case study: Kevin

Kevin is a sensitive, anxious boy with language processing disorder, autism, executive function difficulties and sensory integration problems. Kevin tries hard to co-operate and comply with demands. He works well at imitating movements and has made a lot of progress with co-ordination and rhythm, balance and strengthening exercises. He can manage to choose activities, but relies on familiarity. Kevin enjoys praise and is clearly motivated to become more competent, but is easily overcome if the situation is different from what he is used to, and the challenge is not rightly pitched to his ability to process, plan and physically accomplish; he finds it hard to cope with anything new. He glows with victory when he achieves physical challenges that he sets himself, feeding his self-image.

Familiarity helps him to relax; integrating rhythmic and resistive exercises also help his hypersensitivity. Proprioception in the form of resistive movement exercises and deep touch via the net are helpful for strengthening his experience of his bodily self; these exercises reduce some of his anxiety and his tactile sensitivity.

FROM AN UPDATE REPORT, JANUARY 2010, AGED THIRTEEN

Kevin has attended weekly. Visual aids support his communication.

The exercises include a developmental movement sequence, weight-bearing, activity on suspended equipment (e.g. rings and bar), and balance and co-ordination exercises. Kevin has delicate skin and indicates that he experiences the friction against his hands when using rings or rope, also against his body when doing crawling/creeping exercises, but seems to feel more robust through the experiences of proprioception and has of late been increasing his own intensive activity considerably and with great enjoyment.

Kevin's finer co-ordination skills are growing: catching and throwing rods, crossing the mid-line, balancing while working with smaller balls, playing scoop-ball and throwing balls to target.

Kevin enjoys physical activity, has increased his strength and has fun making efforts, and has come a long way in self-confidence and flexibility. He will benefit from continuing to attend.

From biannual report, January 2011, aged fourteen

Kevin has attended weekly thirty-minute sessions for the last two and a half years.

The aims of the sessions are to give Kevin healthy movement experience, strengthen his proprioception, muscle tone and body scheme, and support bi-lateral integration, differentiation and fine co-ordination.

Kevin clearly enjoys the sessions and makes good use of equipment. His flexibility has increased; he is far less bound by having to follow strict routines. Given choices he tends to go for the well known.

Kevin practices postural exercises, balancing and adaptive responses on suspended equipment and body balls. We also work with rhythm and breathing. Kevin makes excellent efforts and appears to have fun, particularly when challenged with, for example, increased speed.

Sensory issues: Kevin appears easily overwhelmed, and would rather follow than initiate. His hearing is oversensitive. These factors, and stress levels as he struggles to attend to demands, seem to contribute to interference in his ability to concentrate, process language and execute tasks. He has difficulty copying movements, also small movements on paper in the form of writing.

Active fun movement that enhances body feedback seems to help Kevin feel more relaxed and stronger in himself.

Kevin is working hard at trying to speak along with the verse from his own initiative. His arm movements are much improved. He is able to toss and catch the rod while turning his wrist timed to song. His co-ordination is very good: he can turn the rod in spiralling movements round his body while slowly going down to sit on heels and up again on toes; he can toss the rod from hand to hand over his head, and also toss the rod in rhythmic flow between us, passing the rod from left to right.

Co-ordinating feet with arms is more difficult and needs much conscious effort; music helps. Kevin did excellently with proprioceptive stabilising and strengthening exercises: the wave, cradle, plank, bridge, then crab and bear-walk for good measure. After going on the rings and the bar, we did movement exercises in front of the mirror, and Kevin again showed me how, when aware, he can move his arms, wrists and hands with much greater skill than before.

To add, Kevin often took the initiative to set himself big challenges in the 'choose & play' section of the sessions. He would pull himself up onto the large ball with the help of a suspended rope, climb to stand upright, holding onto the rope and balancing, utterly concentrated; then, full of determination and concentration let go of the rope, clap his hands while holding the balance, before dropping to land (with a bounce) seated on the ball, then sliding down to land on his feet on the floor! This was the timid Kevin!

Results of the exercises

What can I see as a result of this work?

Johnny, after developing a strong obsession with me, suddenly chose to stop coming after there had been some change in the timetable. However, I am confident that the work done has been supportive and provided him with one building block in his development; and he may wish to take up an offer of another block next year.

Kevin continues to do very well, and his co-ordination, strength and ability have much developed; he has also grown physically. He can, for example, now co-ordinate his arms and legs very well when doing 'star jumps'; he is much more aware of his arms and hands, his middle is freer, he is also able to tie his shoe laces and plait. He works hard at sounding vowels and other speech exercises. Kevin appears these days far more confident. When meeting him outside school hours, he always greets me with a big smile – before he would have been too overcome by the situation.

Analysis and remediation

Next I will include some points useful for analysing arousal levels, likes, needs and the setting up of an action plan from Sensory Integration literature (source: Murray-Slutsky, Paris 2000).

STEP ONE: ANALYSE THE CHILD'S AROUSAL AND ACTIVITY LEVELS THROUGHOUT THE DAY.

Collect observations and analyse the sensory qualities encountered in two typical days: a structured school or work day, and an unstructured day during the weekend. Record the child's state when he or she gets up in the morning and so on.

Address general questions, for example: During which part of the day is the child most organised? During which part of the day is the child disorganised or showing diminished behaviour or performance? Under what conditions does the child display low arousal levels versus high arousal levels? Are these predictable cycles?

STEP TWO: DEVELOP AN ACTION PLAN BASED ON CAREFUL ANALYSIS OF CHILD'S LIKES, DISLIKES AND NEEDS.

1. Identify the child's likes or needs, factors that contribute to the child's ability to function. This includes:
    ❋ Activities or sensory-based activities that are calming, pleasurable and organising for the child. Identify the activity, if it is socially acceptable.

For activities that are not acceptable or desirable, identify the social component.

᛭ Times and situations in which the child functions optimally and operates in the calm-alert state. Define specific factors that appear to contribute to this.

2. Identify negative factors, activities disliked or avoided, and activities that contribute to sensory overload or shutdown. This includes:

᛭ Times and situations throughout the day in which the child does not function optimally. Define specific factors that contribute to this.

᛭ Environmental factors that have an adverse impact on the child's functional performance and contribute to sensory overload. Consider organisational aspects, sensory components, arousal levels, activity demands, frustration levels created by the activity, and so on.

᛭ Coping strategies that are either not effective or are not socially acceptable for the environment.

3. Establish an action plan.

᛭ Identify several powerful sensory-based activities that are socially acceptable and effective in either raising or lowering the child's level of arousal into the calm-alert state. Determine the length of effectiveness of each activity.

᛭ Establish therapeutic routines to address the child's attention, organisation and arousal levels and to optimise performance. Develop routines that incorporate sensory-based activities, which meet the child's arousal and organisational needs in all daily activities: waking up, dressing, throughout school hours, during transitions, mealtimes, leisure activities, bathing, bedtime, and so on.

❋ Modify the child's environment for optimal state of arousal, and therefore function.

❋ If necessary, teach the child how to perform and use the sensory-based activity in order to derive the sensory experience.

❋ Teach the child self-regulation: to identify signs of escalating behaviours or low arousal levels, and to seek out appropriate sensory-based activities to obtain the optimal arousal level.

❋ Activities geared at increasing the child's arousal level must be used cautiously for a child with a fluctuating or defensive disorder, which results from an unstable and volatile nervous system. Activities that increase the child's arousal level might contribute to the instability of the child's condition. Use activities that incorporate deep-touch and deep-proprioceptive input, and therefore have an impact on the limbic system and the reticular formation of the brain.

Conclusion

It is essential that sensory issues in autism are better understood, and that these issues and their ramifications are taken to heart by the many people involved in supporting people with autism. The senses themselves may work perfectly well, but problems lie in the sifting and processing systems. Such distortions may mean that our autistic friends get an altered perception of the reality we share, for example (some of these are taken from Caldwell 2008):

❋ A room may suddenly change its apparent size.

❋ The straight line between the wall and the floor may wriggle.

❋ People may be unable to sustain their feeling of self when shifting from one space to another.

❀ People may not know where they are in space or even if they are the right way up, becoming anxious when their feet are off the ground.

❀ A shower can feel like red-hot needles jabbing into the skin.

So how can we help? How can we best create an autism friendly environment? How can we communicate meaningfully? How can we facilitate further development and learning, which may well prove to be a mutual path in the end?

The first step is to understand more deeply what our friends may be experiencing, and for that we need to train our observation and open our minds to a different world experience. I would highly recommend reading autistic authors, such as Ros Blackburn, Gunilla Gerland, Temple Grandin, T. Jolliffe, Wendy Lawson and Donna Williams to get first-hand insights into the phenomena of life with autism. I can also warmly recommend reading Phoebe Caldwell for excellent insights and Olga Bogdashina's well-researched books on autism, senses and modes of perception.

9. Intensive Interaction Case Study: Anna

PAULA JACOBS

Intensive interaction (II) is an approach that works on establishing positive experiences of social interactions with people with severe learning difficulties. This assignment arose from my personal experience of how therapeutic play can help to address issues of isolation and withdrawal in children and young adults with autism and severe learning difficulties. In therapeutic play settings, I observed progress in social interactions when therapists used intense interactive approaches, responding to every sign of a possible interaction. Using techniques of II had also helped me to relate to some of our more challenging residents. This chapter will describe and evaluate an intervention using II with an adolescent on the autistic spectrum.

The setting

I work and live in a residential Camphill school for children and young adults with a variety of complex special needs. Most children live on the estate and go to school on campus. They require specialised programmes in which we incorporate elements of education, care, craft and therapies.

I am part of a small team that runs a house of six children and young adults. I also run therapeutic play and II sessions with some of the residents, who are mainly on the autistic spectrum – either one to one or group sessions. I am supervised by a qualified play therapist, who supports me in planning and conducting the sessions. I have a background in social pedagogy, which is a well-established profession in Scandinavia, Germany and Switzerland but is little known in Britain.

179

Cameron and Moss (2011) describe social pedagogy as a place where education and care meet: we follow the ethos that education doesn't only take place in school; learning and teaching are part of everyday life and every moment contains the possibility for development – going for a walk, sharing a meal or socialising in the sitting room. We not only work with the children but we share living space, as many practitioners live on campus or in the houses alongside the students. Social pedagogy believes that relationships are central to the realm of care and education.

Introduction to Anna

Anna is a fourteen-year-old adolescent, resident in the house community where I work. She lives with us during the week, attends school on campus and goes home at weekends. She is nonverbal but can communicate her needs using signs and picture exchange systems (PECS). She responds well to visual cues and likes routines and rituals. Anna is diagnosed with autism, epilepsy and severe learning difficulties.

During an internal review meeting attended by teachers, therapists, a doctor, key-worker and house-coordinator, concerns were raised regarding Anna's progress. After a very settled period she had started to present more challenging behaviour, and it was felt that she was in danger of becoming increasingly isolated. This seemed to arise out of staff changes. I was asked to start sessions of therapeutic play to create an opportunity for Anna to experience social interaction in a positive way.

Intensive interaction

Intensive interaction, developed by Hewett & Nind (2008), is an approach to develop communication and build meaningful relationships with people with communication and severe learning difficulties. It is based on infant-caregiver interactions, such as:

❄ Building a safe environment in which to interact.
❄ Creating an atmosphere of exploration, with no dominance or controlling elements from the caregiver, but an openness and interest for the other's actions.
❄ Responsiveness to every behaviour observed.
❄ Enjoying time together so the child can learn that it's good to be with people.
(Hewett & Nind 2008)

Zeedyk supports the argument that knowledge of infant-mother interactions can help practitioners to interact with people with complex needs. She states, 'The key to establishing, expanding or maintaining the self-awareness of these individuals may be to ensure that, like infants, they first (re-)experience themselves as the undoubted object of another person's attention' (Zeedyk 2006, 328).

Zeedyk (2006) describes early interactions as being characterised by rhythm, turn-taking, anticipation and burst-pause moments. Hence those interactions are very intense as the focus of the other is concentrated, reciprocal and absolute.

The Scottish Intercollegiate Guidelines Network (SIGN 2007) appeals for practitioners to use approaches whose effectiveness is validated by research. At the time of writing, intensive interaction is still a young approach so research is scarce. Most intensive interaction research comes from small-scale studies and or qualitative case studies (Leaning and Watson 2006).

Intensive interaction: a useful approach for ASD?

I would like to evaluate briefly if II is a valid approach for individuals with ASD.

Jordan and Powell (1995) propose how not having Theory of Mind (see Chapter 4, p.89) means that individuals will not initiate social interaction; they will expect other people to know what they want without them needing to communicate it. Hence it is very likely that motivation to initiate will be a problem. II tries to address this by creating moments where the individual finds an interaction so enjoyable, they will want it to happen again; and to do so they will need to communicate this to their partner (Hewett & Nind 2000).

Furthermore, facilitating joint attention (see Chapter 10, p.191) through copying and joining an individual in his or her world of experience is one of the aims of II (Hewett & Nind, 2000). Nind (1996) also argues that interactive approaches are relevant for ASD as they build on infant and mother interactions and use early developmental processes.

Caldwell (2007) states that stereotyped behaviours often have a sensory component, as individuals stimulate a certain sense through their behaviours. Sensory exploration is a big part of II, which considers stereotyped behaviours to be meaningful and a base for interaction (Hewett & Nind 2000). Jordan and Powell (1995) describe how using a child's obsession as a starting point can be an effective way to facilitate learning; not to encourage the obsession but to find a way of engagement.

Ethical considerations: Autism Spectrum Difference

Bogdashina (2006), drawing on experience of individuals with autism, tries to explain how difference is not to be confused with inability. She states that ASD needs to be understood as a different way of perceiving, interpreting and thinking: 'In short ... a fundamentally different way of being' (Bogdashina 2006, 89).

As a practitioner, this presents me with the following question: Do I believe that your social interaction and communication is impaired, or can you and I interact if I join your world?

This is the starting point of intensive interaction described by Caldwell, Hewett and Nind. From an ethical point of view II values all behaviour as meaningful, and it values individuals in a powerful way because it does not attempt to change them. During my sessions I do not try to change Anna, but I start with myself. I make the first step to come closer to Anna.

Sensory assessment

> *Anna sits in the sitting room waiting for lunch. There are ten other people in the room. One boy is chatting excitedly while another one makes loud noises and jumps up and down in his seat. Several co-workers talk about their evening plans.*
>
> *Anna rocks in her chair. She covers her ears with her hands. After a while she throws a shoe then when told off she closes her eyes tightly and crouches down. When called for lunch she is frozen on her chair. After ten minutes she starts to move and crawls to the table.*

I wondered how my attitude towards Anna and assessment of her would change if I considered ASD as a different way of being instead of a disorder? Bogdashina (2006) claims that it would lead to a different interpretation of the behaviours observed. Considering it and reflecting on my talks with colleagues, I realised how much our attitudes and our views on autism influence our practice. Looking back on the description of Anna waiting for lunch, I can see how my reaction to the situation makes a difference: if I think she throws her shoe to be annoying, I tell her off, reacting merely to her behaviour; if I think that the noise and movement around her probably cause her pain and distress, I can understand why she throws the shoe and I can try to reduce the sensory stimuli around her. I began to wonder: if we as practitioners want to change our practice, do we need to change our attitudes first?

With the help of Anna's parents, school and her key-worker, I completed Bogdashina's sensory profile (see Chapter 8, p.161), which led us to conclude the following about Anna's sensory experiences: Anna seems to take in most information using vision and hearing. Her vision seems to be her strength. She seems to think visually and make sense of the world using visual clues. However, there seems to be vulnerability to sensory overload for vision, hearing and a possibility of gestalt perception, which can lead to system shutdowns. Her smell and taste senses don't suggest unusual experiences.

However, looking at her tactile, proprioception and vestibular systems, a picture of uncertainty emerged. She seems to experience sensory input in a delayed, distorted and fragmented way. This fitted well with my knowledge of Anna. She is a very observant young woman, noticing small changes and details. She likes to watch rather than to engage in an activity. Her experience of the three senses that connect to movement seem to be fragmented or delayed. This could explain her difficulties in engagement. For example, it might explain her freezing in the situation described earlier.

From the sensory assessment and our following group discussion, I drew these conclusions for the implementation of my sessions:

1. To build on Anna's strengths: structure our session room visually and use big pictures.
2. To encourage movement and tactile interactions.

My intervention is part of a holistic programme. Anna also uses PECs, visual timetables and has music and movement therapy. Humphrey & Parkinson (2006) state how combined elements of PECs, visual timetables, intensive interaction and behavioural approaches have proven very successful.

Hence my sessions are not aimed to address all of Anna's needs alone but they should complement her other approaches and interventions. I decided to use PECs within my sessions as Anna is used to using them in other settings.

Implementation

Anna wraps a rubbery toy around her hand while rocking back and forth. I join in with her rocking, take a similar toy and start to copy her. She watches me, makes eye contact for a few seconds, smiles and then drops the toy on the ground. I drop my toy too. She looks at me again and smiles excitedly. She then points at my toy. I pass it to her and she takes it. She withdraws eye contact and continues to engage in her play.

Anna is not only diagnosed with ASD but also with epilepsy and learning difficulties. Jordan (2005) states that the combination of lack of cognitive underpinning and impairment of social interaction means that interactions become more difficult. Hence Jordan sees a priority in helping the individual to develop an understanding of what communication is.

For our sessions this meant that in the beginning I would provide Anna with a choice of toys and objects. She could choose a preferred activity and through this activity I would try to find ways of engaging with her, starting with the early forms of communication: joint attention.

I started our five sessions on the November 7, and they took place in the morning in a small room at school. Building on my sensory assessment, I divided our room into different corners: one for tactile toys; one for musical instruments; one to lie down and relax; one for teddies; and one for matching and sorting activities.

Anna seemed to respond well to the sessions. She came along and engaged in different activities for short amounts of time. To facilitate joint attention, I joined Anna in her games. As described in the extract above, she noticed me and we shared attention during our play with the rubbery toy.

I enjoyed the sessions very much and it helped me to see Anna in a different light. Now I can see her as someone who is curious and particularly enjoys interactions of anticipation and burst-pause interactions.

Zeedyk (2006) argues that the intimacy between two people within an interaction is the base for all future learning. I started to realise that this does not only include Anna's learning, but mine as well. Becoming more attuned to Anna means that I feel more confident to be with her outside our sessions; I am learning to read her behaviour better.

As described in the extract, Anna initiated eye contact during our sessions and was able to engage in turn-taking interactions for short periods of time. Anna enjoys anticipation, e.g. blowing up a balloon, waiting for a few seconds and then letting it go. She can easily get overwhelmed and then withdraws for a short period before she is able to interact again. Trying to expand the time she can stay engaged will be one of my future aims.

Considering those five sessions I argue that II does help Anna to engage in social interactions. Deepening my knowledge of ASD, especially with regard to sensory experiences and joint attention, has helped me to plan our sessions in accordance with Anna's needs.

I also agree with Hewett & Nind (2008), who claim that II is not exclusively for people with ASD. It is designed for individuals with severe learning and communication difficulties, which applies to most people with ASD but also to those with other complex needs.

Reflection

Anna is in the swimming pool with her key-worker. She splashes water and watches the drops. Her key-worker splashes some water too. They continue to take turns splashing and watching the other one a few more times. Anna moves towards her key-worker, takes her hands and smiles. Her key-worker pulls her gently around the water while talking quietly to her.

After two sessions with Anna, I talked to her key-worker. She seemed excited to hear how it was going and interested in learning new ways of interacting with Anna. One aspect of her feedback was especially interesting to me. She said how nice it was to see someone else taking an interest and enjoying time with Anna. This again made me aware of the importance of collaborative practice and how we can inspire each other. I started to observe how their interactions had become playful and attuned to one another, as described in the extract above. To be able to use II techniques, you need to be open to joining the residents in their world. One of the biggest challenges for me personally was to be able to let Anna lead the interactions, and regular reflections on my own behaviour with my supervisor helped my development.

However, when considering the implications of this intervention for Anna's life in a wider context, I found it difficult to imagine future steps. Our school has many young co-workers with little training, some of whom I supervise. After our talks, I often come back to the importance of attitudes. Just recently I challenged a colleague to use more visual support when communicating with one of the residents.

I explained that the resident found it difficult to relate to spoken language; not reacting to instructions didn't mean that he was acting up, but simply that he didn't understand. During the next few days I did not observe an increase in the use of visual symbols or hand gestures. I think this is because the co-worker could not imagine the resident's way of being as different from his own.

Firth, Elford, *et al.* (2007) did a study into care staff's views on II. They found that it was difficult for many to understand that changes in their behaviour could help students make more sense of interactions. Preformed conceptions of students' abilities, not based on actual assessments, were also found to be an obstacle in using II. For example, one staff member described a client as non-tactile who was later found to enjoy tactile play.

Furthermore, some staff members had not acknowledged that most behaviours, vocalisation or stereotypical play could have communicative intent. The described reluctance to change connects to Bogdashina's (2006) call for an addition to the Theory of Mind: a Theory of Autistic Minds (ToAM). We say that 'they' find it difficult to read 'our' minds, and Bogdashina goes on to question if 'we' find it easy to understand 'their' minds. Reflecting on my experience as a supervisor and someone working with individuals with ASD, I agree: don't we lack a Theory of Autistic Minds?

Richter and Coates (2001) stress that with autism comes the difficulty not only for them to reach out, but for us to reach into their world. I think it is important for us to realise this. Anna and I have the best interactions when I am fully attuned to her. To be attuned means that I give my full attention to her, leaving behind my own needs and expectations. It sounds easy, but it is often very difficult not to let my need for achievement get in the way. In such moments I react too quickly and don't give Anna enough time. Learning about attunement requires the ability for self-reflection and awareness of our own needs (Feilberg 2009). Hence I believe that it is important to create spaces for self-reflection through supervision, videoing or working groups.

Considering my intervention from an institutional point of view, II training could help staff to find new ways of relating and interacting with residents. I have also learned that finding out more about the influence of personal values and beliefs on practice might be very helpful for my own sessions and my work with colleagues.

II accepts individuals with their special interests and, considering that it starts with the practitioner rather than the individual changing, I think it is a very interesting approach. Changing ourselves sounds simple, but in my experience it is very difficult. It is a highly complex topic, which touches on issues of power and control within care settings, but I think it is worth being more aware of in the future.

10. Art Club Case Study: Ralph, Mark and Oliver

RÉKA TÓTH

This chapter examines and evaluates a creative group activity called the Art Club as a social intervention for learners on the autism spectrum. It considers three individuals who participate in a weekly Art Club, all of whom have a diagnosis of autism spectrum disorder with additional learning difficulties. The Art Club is based upon art therapy principles, and is specifically designed to accommodate the learning needs of these individuals.

Setting

I work in a residential Camphill school for children with additional support needs. Most of the carers, teachers and other professionals are volunteers and share the living space with the learners. The institution has three main areas: house life (care), school and therapies. Based on individual needs the learners have day, weekly or full-time placements. The mission statement of the school describes the basic principles and values of the organisation: '...it aims to create a community in which vulnerable children and adults, many with learning disability, can live, learn and work with others in healthy social relationships based on mutual care and respect'.
(Chepelina *et al.* 2009)

These principles can also be seen through theories of social pedagogy. Most members of our schools are trained social pedagogues. The underlying ideology of social pedagogy is based on the understanding of each child from a holistic perspective, which acknowledges individual uniqueness and needs. All individuals are supported in their overall development. Practitioners share life space with the learners. Professional development is based on collaborative practice and self-reflection. The ability to listen, communicate and reflect is the basis of relationship building, which is one of the central aspects of social pedagogy (Cameron and Moss 2011).

Ralph, Mark and Oliver

During this study, there were four members of the group, and my focus will be directed towards the three learners diagnosed with ASD: Mark, Ralph and Oliver.

Mark and Ralph attend the sessions with their helpers and Oliver participates individually. Due to their diagnoses and individual abilities, all three learners find social interaction challenging at times. Ralph and Mark have no speech and Oliver has limited verbal language. While Ralph can be very vocal in social settings, Mark and Oliver might find auditory stimuli overwhelming. They all show behaviours that indicate extreme awareness towards their environment. All learners display repetitive behaviours and patterns of thought, which increases when uncertainty is experienced, and may lead to extreme anxiety. Therefore providing routine and structure is essential in order to create a predictable and secure learning environment.

All learners seem to be very interested in creating art. They show high levels of motivation when the right level of activity is provided. I wonder if they enjoy using glue, paper, clay and paints out of tactile experience, or if they enjoy watching the objects and the visual marks they create. I classify interest and motivation as positive feedback.

All learners have been referred to the Art Club to address individual needs in a group setting. Mark joined the Art Club with the aim of experiencing peer interaction outside the class while working with creative materials. Ralph's target is to develop skills that will help him to learn and interact in group settings. Oliver's aim is to participate independently in a group activity; he is encouraged to take part in practical tasks in order to develop flexible thinking, redirecting his thinking from fixed patterns of ideas.

The Art Club and art therapy

The Art Club is a weekly afternoon lesson, designed with a specific aim of having fun using creativity and art materials. I am not a trained art therapist, but providing therapeutic art activities was the focus of my social pedagogy degree. I am independently in charge of planning and implementing all activities. The Art Club is a creative activity, based upon art therapy principles, but it is not group art therapy.

Art therapy is a wide field with various different approaches. Practitioners agree about the therapeutic effect of the authentic creative process. However, there are various views about purpose, methods and expectations of art therapy (Osborne 2003; Rubin 2001). In order to give a detailed picture of my practice in theoretical context, I will focus on autism specific art-therapy theories.

Art therapy as an autism intervention aims to promote change and growth on a personal level through self-expression, which allows the learner to adapt to the social world in the safe and facilitated environment of the art room. Through working with art materials, such as painting, drawing, pottery and craft, a positive social experience is created. This is the basis of relationship development between learner and therapist (Bragge & Fenner 2009; Research Autism 2012).

Art therapy and joint attention development

The triadic exchange between infant, mother and their co-ordinated attention around an object is called joint attention. It develops from early interaction between mother and child, involving gestures, eye-contact and the awareness of shared experiences (Baron-Cohen *et al.* 1993; Hobson 1993). However Baron Cohen *et al* and Hobson propose that infants with ASD do not develop joint attention skills.

A similar triadic exchange can be established between therapists and learners by paying attention to and creating an art object, opening up a space for social engagement and shared experiences. In art therapy, this is the basis of positive relationship development between learner and therapist (Isserow 2008).

I therefore wonder if the triangle of art therapy can be comprehended as an alternative approach to address joint attention difficulties. Instead of focusing on the dyadic relationship development between therapist and learner (which in this case is compared to the mother and child interaction), the focus is on co-ordinating attention around an art object. In addition, visual art provides shared experiences through reciprocal movements, gestures and sensory experiences, which are more similar to pre-verbal communication between mother and child (Osborne 2003).

Furthermore, I wonder if the triadic relationship development between learner and therapist can be translated to developing relationships between peers at the Art Club, fostered by relating and interacting via each other's artwork. An alternative means of dialogue is established, which is believed to be beneficial for learners with ASD, who tend to withdraw from direct focus and expectation of establishing social connections (Isserow 2008). Learners at the Art Club also establish shared experiences through copying each other's work, sharing material and presenting their art to the rest of the group.

In summary, the visual and creative process in a tactile domain can potentially enhance the establishment of social structures and common language based on shared experiences (Osborne 2003; Emery & Forest 2004; Isserow 2008). Shared experiences must be established before joint attention can develop (Isserow 2008; Bragge & Fenner 2009). Therefore I am convinced that the Art Club is a successful social intervention for these three learners with ASD.

Implementation and observation

I observed three sessions, in order to identify ways to enhance learning skills and develop peer interaction in the group environment.

Session 1

The aim of Session 1 was to illustrate the present stage of the group regarding the introduction of a new craft activity. We made paper lanterns using scissors, crayons and rulers. We had not used rulers before in this setting. Each learner showed a high level of participation and interest. They were all focused and calm. It was a positive social experience for everyone. The design of the paper lantern activity was based on my knowledge of the learners' individual interests (e.g. using glue sticks and crayons). Consequently, a fun activity was provided whilst individual targets were addressed by learning new skills (using the ruler) in a group setting. This was also a practical activity, which encouraged peer interaction.

Session 2

Taking Session 1 into consideration I designed an activity that provided another opportunity for using rulers. We made heart-shaped paper decorations.

Individual aims were addressed by encouraging peer interaction via sharing material and tools.

In Session 2 all learners used the ruler independently according to their potential. Therefore I conclude that all learners were able to internalise a new skill when it was introduced in a familiar setting and opportunities of practice were provided.

In summary of the evaluation of the first two Art Club sessions, I concluded that all learners were able to focus, follow instructions and learn new skills in this specific group environment. However I noticed that all learners followed my instructions very well but had little opportunity to initiate or express their opinion or preferences during the activities. Oliver has limited verbal commutation and Mark and Ralph have no speech, but in spite of this I strongly believe they hold opinions regarding the activities.

It is also acknowledged in the Scottish national guideline for ASD (SLD *et al.* 2009) that all individuals with ASD have opinions, although they might have particular barriers for expressing them. Consequently I had to consider how to provide opportunities for the learners to give feedback on their educational programme, and support them to express their opinions in my practice setting. I found this issue exceptionally complicated as all three learners have limited communication. However, behaviour can be understood as a form of communication (Shaddock *et al.* 2000). Therefore structured observation was needed to create the best possible interpretation of the behaviour (SLD *et al.* 2009).

I concluded that all three learners were able to express their like or dislike of the art activity through their behaviour, and that identifying enhanced ways of communication to express opinions and preferences was a learning need of the Art Club group.

Introducing PECS: requests and preferences

Based on my practice and theoretical knowledge, I believed that enhanced visual communication via visual symbols and picture exchange communication systems (PECS) would address the aim of allowing individuals to initiate and express preferences. Hence, to obtain best practice I was faced with the following questions: why is PECS beneficial for all learners? Is the Art Club a suitable setting to introduce PECS? What is the best way to use visual symbols and PECS at the Art Club?

PECS was originally designed to teach functional communication skills for individuals with little or no language with ASD (Roth 2010; Sulzer-Azaroff *et al.* 2009). PECS has been evaluated in various efficacy studies, and has been identified as one of the few scientifically proven widely beneficial ASD interventions (ibid; Boucher 2009). At the present moment Ralph and Mark only uses PECS at mealtimes to request food. The use of PECS at the Art Club would be an opportunity to extend this communication skill, and further encourage more complex communication, such as comments on what one sees (ibid; Roth 2010).

Conclusively the use of visual symbols and PECS is potentially beneficial for all learners at the Art Club. Initially I identified the aim of requesting objects, like glue and scissors, which later on could be developed to express preferences between activities such as painting or drawing.

Session 3

The aim of Session 3 was to introduce the use of PECS and large visual symbols in the Art Club setting. The individual assessment sheets clearly demonstrated improved focus, independence and participation. To my surprise Mark and Ralph used their PECS folders with ease appropriately and independently. Oliver followed the activity independently and clearly benefited from the visual support of step-by-step introduction.

All learners benefited from the use of visual support. I believe the use of PECS not only encouraged Ralph and Mark to request objects, but enabled them to participate more actively. Consequently the use of PECS and visual symbols enhanced independent participation and peer interaction, through establishing a common language between all participants, which seemed to support all learners to be more secure and confident in this setting. The use of visual communication enabled the Art Club to become a better learning environment for the learners.

Strengths and limitations of the Art Club as a social intervention

Based on the theoretical discussion of the triangular relationship-building process between therapist and learners, and the successful implementation of PECS to enhance learning skills and peer interaction, I propose that the Art Club is a successful social intervention.

However, I must state that there is very little empirical evidence that any form of art therapy is a successful intervention for ASD (Humphrey & Parkinson 2006; Research Autism 2012). Most professional research is based on small-scale studies without a comparison group, which leads to difficulties in creating a general picture due to the heterogeneity of the condition (Jones & Jordan 2008; Humphrey & Parkinson 2006). All theoretical data I have referred to in this assignment regarding art therapy as an autism specific intervention was based on either a single case study (Emery & Forest 2004) or a series of case studies without a comparison group (Bragge & Fenner 2009; Isserow 2008). Therefore, I wonder if the validity of creating a general picture of art therapy as an intervention can be questioned. Consequently, I agree with Martin (2009), who claims that art therapy has the potential to be a successful intervention for ASD via addressing individual needs through visual communication, socialisation and sensory regulation. However, in order to provide empirical research evidence to validate this approach, the focus needs to be directed towards quantitative data, larger sample groups and comparative studies.

11. Ways Forward

Using Steiner's Image of Man

The way in which we have come to understand childhood autism in this book has evolved over time, based firmly on anthroposophy's Image of Man. This image is multifaceted and differentiated, and yet forms a holistic and consistent totality. Centrally, it takes into account the fundamental human threefoldness of body, soul and spirit, and of the relationships of these realities to the physical, material world on one hand, and the spiritual, non-material world on the other. The human soul as intermediary is the dynamic scenario where influences from both spheres of existence mix and mingle, and it is here that experiences unfold, both in the drama of daily existence and in the course of our individual biographical development.

In any comparison of the anthroposophic interpretation of autism with other mainstream explanations, it is essential to try to identify exactly which model of the human being underpins the explanation. Furthermore, within any particular model it may be possible to focus at different levels, such as the biological or psychological (Happé 1994). Clearly, different interpretations of autism are likely to emerge from a predominantly biological or behavioural model of man, as compared to a largely psychodynamic perception in which the importance of inner soul-states and dynamic relationships between people is emphasised.

The anthroposophic model is inclusive, rather than one-sidedly exclusive. It fully recognises the level of biological processes (underpinned by the physical and etheric organisation), and also the psychological levels of consciousness within the soul (underpinned by the etheric, and especially the astral organisation). In addition, it acknowledges the spiritual level (underpinned by the ego), on which we encounter the unique being of ourselves and others.

We have argued in this book that a holistic, anthroposophic perspective can provide a more complete understanding of autism than is to be found at the present time in mainstream literature, which emphasises the biological, organic view of autism. This view is, however, not contradicted by the anthroposophic perspective, provided that the organic is seen as one level of explanation, and is not accepted as the be all and end all.

The same proviso applies if we focus on the child's cognitive faculties at the psychological level, as has been done by Theory of Mind researchers (see Chapter 4, p.89 and Chapter 9, p. 181), who suggest that children with autism often appear to be mind-blind with regard to their own minds, and to the minds of others (Astington 1994). The anthroposophic model can throw light on this particular problem through an understanding of the differentiated functioning of the four higher senses. However, through anthroposophy we do not only encompass a variety of different levels within the human being, but also, and more importantly, we are led to a recognition of the child's essential being. The child's individual spiritual being (the ego) is not sufficiently, if at all, acknowledged by mainstream models of man, not even on the psychodynamic level (Lievegoed 1993). It is precisely the awareness of the real being of the child that underpins curative education, and the wide choice of interventions this generates. Therefore, the Image of Man gives us the necessary spiritual-scientific foundation for new ways of both understanding and alleviating autism.

New avenues of research

> There is no known cure for autism, and indeed a search
> for a cure may well be misguided because it is not a
> sickness in any simple sense, but our knowledge of its
> causes and how to intervene to help the child and family
> is growing rapidly in a period of unprecedented research
> activity and public interest. (Trevarthen *et al.* 1996, 3)

The anthroposophic interpretation of autism, and the attitudes and interventions that curative education makes available, deserve to be fully included in this current and on-going research work. There is an urgent need to critically examine the uniqueness of the anthroposophic contribution. However, it requires further study and research to describe and investigate in detail the physiology, functioning, genesis and development of the total sense organism. The developmental correspondences between the four higher and the four lower senses, which are clearly an essential component in the anthroposophic interpretation of autism, could constitute an extensive and exciting new research area. As König (1984) indicated, we have hardly begun to explore thoroughly, or to differentiate between the three higher senses of word, thought and ego that Steiner originally described (1981 & 1990b).

Another area that begs investigation, and which is central to the anthroposophic model, is the development of typical self-cognition in young children. Only when this is more thoroughly understood will we be better able to confirm the importance of that inner awakening to the self, and to self-referencing through language: 'It is not yet possible to provide an adequate account of early "self"-development in autistic children...' (Hobson 1993, 76).

Such an account would be of central importance to the understanding of the asocial behaviours of these children. Linked to this theme of self-cognition is the child's sensitive peripheric awareness, which generally calls for an indirect and gentle therapeutic approach. More generally, the nature of cognition and thinking in relation to the development of self should certainly be examined further: 'Just as the colour-blind see only differences of brightness without colour qualities, so someone who lacks intuition sees only unconnected perceptible fragments' (Steiner 1992, 64). Steiner's remark is indicative of the situation in which children with autism so often find themselves. This appears to be clearly corroborated by autobiographical accounts of recovering individuals with autism, who have struggled to make coherent sense of their sensory perceptions (Grandin 1986; Williams 1992).

Yet another essential research theme that autism highlights is an investigation into the deeper nature and important developmental role of imitation: 'The first thing to note is the general agreement that autistic children demonstrate abnormal delay and limitation in their imitation of others' (Hobson 1993, 73). As we showed in Chapter 4, this delay and limitation is evidence of the lack of early ego-integration and individualisation in these children.

Finally, an area that urgently warrants special attention is that of how to arrive at exact differential diagnoses, with correspondingly appropriate curative educational measures, for primary and secondary forms of autism. Sahlmann's (1969) initial observations and research into the identification and treatment of children who have a secondary autism due to an underlying primary aphasia should be developed further. In this respect it is not sufficient, either diagnostically or in terms of effective individual interventions, to simply place a child on the broad autistic spectrum, without also making specific reference to any other accompanying disabilities or impairments (Wing 1993).

From the previous chapters, it is clear that the anthroposophic model of autism generates important avenues for valuable research, including practical implementations in the variety of curative educational interventions. Although curative centres aim to provide an integrated holistic environment, this does not mean that the effects of specific types of intervention cannot be investigated and monitored. Clearly, it is important to develop this kind of evaluative research so that clearer differentiations of progress, in relation to specific measures, can be seen. One obvious difficulty in ascertaining the effectiveness of a specific intervention, when conducted over six months or even longer, is to know to what degree natural processes of maturation have contributed to any progress. Therefore when specific interventions, such as eurythmy therapy, art therapy or lower sense exercises, can be implemented intensively over comparatively short periods of time, with the child's responses clearly monitored, it should be much easier to evaluate their effectiveness. However, the specific relationship between child and educator in curative education is a central and inclusive factor in whatever therapy or intervention is employed.

Moral issues

The whole subject of interventions, whether anthroposophic or otherwise, is based on a fundamental assumption that it is justifiable, and indeed morally right, to try to alleviate and, if at all possible, cure autism. This assumption is implicitly underpinned by the notion that the differences children with autism exhibit in their behaviour are deviant from normal children, and socially unacceptable. It follows, therefore, that we should do everything possible to socialise and normalise these children, and this necessitates some form of intervention. Exactly what type of intervention may be applied to a particular child depends upon a number of factors: the latest fashion, parents' perceptions and understanding of their child, the resources on offer etc. See Chapter 5 for explanations of some of the interventions currently used. The book *Cutting-Edge Therapies for Autism* by Siri & Lyons is published every year, and explains different approaches, which have not necessarily been tested.

We could, however, question this whole line of thinking and, from an ethical and anthroposophic perspective, ask if there are deeper reasons for wanting to change children with autism than the goal of *normalisation*.

Rudolf Steiner questioned the whole notion of *normality* when speaking of the child's observable life of soul expressed in its various behaviours.

> This life of soul, which can show itself in varied
> expressions and manifestations, may be normal or it may
> be abnormal. But now the only possible grounds we can
> have for speaking of the normality or abnormality of
> the child's life of soul, or indeed of the life of soul of any
> human being, is that we have in mind something that is
> normal in the sense of being average. There is no other
> criterion than the one that is customary among people
> who abide by ordinary conventions... (Steiner 1972, 17)

Steiner then pointed out that when people apply this criterion, based entirely on what is average or typical, they may readily intervene with children who have been judged as *abnormal*.

> When they have in this way ascertained the existence of 'abnormality', they begin to do – heaven knows what! – believing they are thereby helping to get rid of the abnormality, while all the time they are driving out a fragment of genius! (Steiner 1972, 17)

Steiner goes on:
> We shall get nowhere at all by applying this kind of criterion, and the first thing the doctor and teacher have to do is to reject it and get beyond the stage of making pronouncements as to what is clever or reasonable, in accordance with the habits of thought that prevail today. (Steiner 1972, 17)

I have quoted Steiner at length to show that he did not accept the concept of superficial normalisation, seen in terms of individuals conforming to expected, average standards of behaviour.

Steiner claimed that any interventions must be thoroughly grounded on a deepened understanding of child development that goes far beyond superficial observations and judgments. Therefore, he described the nature of the child's real spiritual being; the processes of incarnation into the threefold bodily organisation; the individualisation of the child's model, inherited body; and even spoke of karmic necessities and reincarnation.

Steiner repeatedly emphasised the moral tenor that should underlie any interventional methods, and educators were called upon to have reverence and respect for the child's real being above all else. In a sense, the child's own being could tell them what needed to be done, in each individual case, but this required educators to consciously develop their powers of empathy.

As our understanding and appreciation of the experience of people with autism grows and deepens, for example, helped by biographical accounts (Williams 1992 and 1994; Grandin 1986; Barron 1993; Sellin 1995), so our own judgments and expectations can change considerably and positively. Some high-functioning people with autism, such as Temple Grandin, realised that autism gave them extra perceptual possibilities, and became quite at ease with their condition once they had learned to live with it.

Developing relationships

A purely organic explanation of autism, which puts the source of the problem firmly in the child, is unlikely to do justice to the role of relationships in contributing to the degree of autism seen in different situations with a particular child. The case studies included in this book clearly indicate that increased contact and communication was achieved through the implementation of curative educational attitudes and exercises that recognised the inner dynamics between educator and child – thus achieving a reduction in autism.

One of the most difficult aspects of living with these children is their seeming indifference and disaffection. This is particularly poignant for those who have a close family connection with them, as is apparent in published parental accounts (Hocking 1990; Kaufman 1976; Lovell 1978). The educator must search for deeper reasons for the child's behaviour, while maintaining a definite warmth of soul and respect for the child.

Steiner gave specific indications and guidelines for the self-education of the educator, to enable them to develop relationships of the right ethical and moral quality: 'So long as the teacher meets the situation with any kind of bias, so long as it can arouse in him irritation or excitement – so long will he remain incapable of making any real progress with the child' (Steiner 1972, 41).

Instead of inner irritation towards the child's difficulties or responses, the educator has to develop a conscious calmness and composure so that the phenomenon he encounters becomes an objective picture. 'Once this has come about, the teacher is there by the side of the child in a true relationship and will do all else that is needful more or less rightly' (Steiner 1972, 41).

The despair, frustration and disappointment a child with autism can arouse within someone who wants to help underlines the considerable challenge posed by the type of rigorous self-education Steiner expected curative educators to pursue.

The development of new relationships is furthered by the holistic context in which curative education is practised, especially in residential centres. The relationships between children with different social abilities is often of great therapeutic value and benefit. While this might perhaps also be seen in schools that only cater for children with autism, the exacerbation of the autistic environment that is inevitably formed by such specialised provision may not be able to generate the diversity and social enrichment available in a more holistic setting. This is not a criticism of the special relationships educators can form with their pupils in schools specifically for children with autism, but simply contrasts the differing environmental resources on offer.

A path of knowledge

Anthroposophy, as presented by Rudolf Steiner in his books and lectures, is described as a path of knowledge. It calls upon those who meet it to begin to actively exercise their own faculties of knowledge. Although a critical and questioning mind is certainly required in studying anthroposophic literature, careful self-observation is also needed to guard against the limitations and narrowness of perception resulting from preconceived notions and prejudices. An openness for something new and perhaps unusual at first sight is required even of the seasoned scholar.

Anthroposophy is neither a religion nor a new faith. It is a spiritual-scientific way of coming to a new and detailed understanding of evolving human beings, and their relationship with the evolving universe. Spiritually, both mankind and our planet are viewed as intimately and inextricably linked in their past and future developments (Steiner 1989).

Autistic behaviour and state of mind are distinct from the person's real, spiritual being. This holds true for us all. We only express our spiritual being through the possibilities we have in this life, defined by gender, race, culture, upbringing and age. We all express our intentions within the remit of our earthly life; this is the challenge and beauty of being human. It is possible that autism is exactly what a person wants to bring to this life at this moment in time.

The knowledge anthroposophy provides enables us to properly acknowledge the real and intact being of each child and this, in itself, is the most far-reaching therapeutic intervention. Through it, children receive both support and encouragement to face the challenges of their earthly existence, painful and difficult as they often are.

Autism is a condition that requires endless patience, baffles us, requires collaboration between professionals and parents, asks the utmost of our love, patience and insight, trust and creativity. It asks the utmost of humanity. No machines, computer programmes or technology will cure it, only endless human attention infused with deep understanding and knowing empathy. Autism therefore calls forth in all the people who work in this field a deep surging for true humanity based on objective love.

Anthroposophy gives a cognitive and holistic perspective which, when implemented in curative education, may eventually enable many more children or adults with autism to discover what Donna Williams (1994) felt to be the most important thing she had learned – AUTISM IS NOT ME!

IV.

SOURCE MATERIAL FROM
HANS MÜLLER-WIEDEMANN

12. Early Diagnosis and Practical Advice for Parents

The following text is taken from a lecture given to paediatricians in Brixen, Italy, on 5 September 1980. First published in the journal Kinderpsychotherapie, *Volume 4, Biermann, Munich, 1981.*

Part One

Early diagnosis of autistic children, and the resulting therapeutic attitudes and curative educational efforts, depend essentially on the initial assumptions under which the diagnostic conclusions of the case history and the observations are made. Kanner and Eisenberg viewed early childhood autism as a developmental disturbance of the emotions, emphasising aspects of communication. Other investigations and theories have been undertaken in the medical-psychological realm, which infer that autism is caused by cognitive disturbances, which can ultimately be traced back to insufficient brain function. As a result, behavioural therapy is directed at the modification of symptoms. However, the biography of the child and their parents is not taken into account.

Another, psychotherapeutical approach, presented primarily by Bettelheim (1967), Ekstein (1973) and Mahler (1968), investigated the manner in which autistic children first of all communicate with their human environment, or rather, how their communication is disturbed in this respect.

In anthroposophic curative education, autistic children are regarded as possessing serious problems in their relationships with the earthly world, which occur immediately after birth. According to Rudolf Steiner's Science of the Senses our perception of the world, which continues to develop after birth, differentiates itself into the experiences of one's own body, surroundings and specifically human environment. In these three areas the autistic child suffers from disturbed development, and the symptoms that appear early on can express themselves in severe symbiotic disturbances, as well as in fixations with respect to conditions of time and space. There is always a marked disturbance in the use of language, which is independent of the levels of semantic or syntactic abilities.

In normal child development, every perception is directed towards the child, through knowledge gained by being able to communicate with other people, mainly through the use of language, including nonverbal language. This facility, however, appears largely unavailable to autistic children.

Interviews with parents regarding their own experiences around the time of conception show that disturbed communication with the child is central to a diagnosis of early childhood autism. Often we hear the mother saying that before the birth she had the curious feeling that her relationship with the child was disturbed, and that this feeling developed only after she had felt the child move in the womb. Other mothers report that throughout the pregnancy they had looked forward to the birth, but that afterwards a marked and unexpected lack of relationship followed, often accompanied by an inexplicable fear regarding the future of the child.

These comments reveal the fact that, even before birth, a child has a soul-spiritual relationship with the mother, and that this relationship, after birth, adapts for new, earthly life conditions.

It is crucial to picture the important and dramatic character of this extraordinary change in the incarnation process of the child after birth, in order to understand and assess the symptoms of autistic children.

We shall never understand autistic children if we start from the viewpoint that they are born as 'a blank page' and that after birth their human-cultural behaviour is merely imprinted on to them.

Where the adaptation towards an earthly sensory world does not sufficiently occur, mothers often report, as one of their earliest observations, that children *looked through* them, did not see them at all, so mothers experienced themselves as not perceived by their children. On the other hand, children, in the course of their development, made use of their mothers in an external sense, as if encountering a useful object. These experiences of interrupted symbiosis are early indications of an autistic syndrome.

I should like to leave the question of the cause of autism open, and to proceed with the description of some of the aspects of early symptoms. We should remember that the symptoms described are not the illness itself, but point to a communication disturbance. Children develop symptoms in order to *survive* their earthly environment, and at the same time call on us to further their maturing of the senses therapeutically. The analysis of sense perceptions, as described by Rudolf Steiner, directs us to begin with the development of the perception of our own body. In the first year of life, normal children acquire an experience of self, through the upright position, by orienting themselves in the forces of gravity and through their own movement. This existential experience of their own life enables children to constitute a world of objects and a shared world of the *you*. For autistic children already in the first sensory motor phase, the individual relationship with a key person, usually the mother, fails to appear, and their attention is directed mainly towards the spatial world.

Active eye contact is disturbed in the first months, or breaks off intermittently later in life, when children are approached and addressed.

Autistic children are often strikingly quiet, do not cry and do not convey their needs, or they demonstrate fear when touched, looked at, or when moved quickly. This can sometimes be seen when nappies need changing, and early gestures that typically accompany daily communication between mother and child may not appear.

There is also an absence of curiosity of gaze, of movements of the head and hands. Invitations to imitate do not flow into the movement-organism of the child, and autistic children show anomalies very early on, revealing that reflex behaviour is not developing sufficiently.

By contrast, there is an extreme sensitivity to impressions of movement close by, and to acoustic, visual and tactile stimuli.

The change to earthly nourishment shows signs of early disturbances, even if the child first accepts the mother's breast: resistance to
chewing solid food; phases of constipation; avoiding eye contact when
being nursed and when taking nourishment; and compulsive staring
at objects instead of the person concerned. From early on only special
foodstuffs are accepted and others are rejected.

The adaption to culturally-provided rhythms of taking nourishment,
turning to another person and seeking care, is usually delayed early
on, and for a long time. Autistic children have difficulty entering into
circadian rhythms, which results in disturbances of the sleeping/
waking rhythm.

Furthermore, it is striking in the first year that children do not
explore objects and usually do not seek contact by mouth. Later,
the exploratory and constructive attitude to play does not occur.
Activities of touching and grasping do not develop progressively,
children become *spectators*, lets others act for them and alternate these
states with chaotic phases of excitement, especially when too much is
demanded of them.

Between the second and third year new symptoms occur, mostly
related to the fact that autistic children do not succeed, or only partly,
in making the world objective; that is, one of objects. Instead, the
world of objects remains only a part of the insufficiently structured
bodily experiences of the child.

This shows, above all, in the area of language where children's
efforts at speech do not develop into a language of meaning (Ekstein
1980, 102–19). The insufficient objectivity of the world extinguishes
the indicating function of language as a decisive medium of increasing
communication. As an expression of this, children's first use of
echolalia appears. Children do not establish ego-consciousness *vis-
à-vis* the non-ego of the world of objects, and do not experience
themselves as speaking individuals, even when they do speak.
Imitation or the beginnings of play do not develop and, at this stage,
the first fear caused by change usually starts to appear. This tends
to happen when children are anxious to set up or keep to the same
spatial arrangements. A lack of orientation also arises with regard to

212

happenings in time, demonstrating a disturbed living experience of time.

No habits of communication are formed with reference to common rhythms of life, and this in particular leads to the first serious burdens on the family.

Phases of being absent, alternating with restlessness or compulsive fixation on certain objects, appear increasingly around the age of three. The lack of further development in movement by not imitating now causes stereotypical movements to appear, which are not related to the environment. Paths of successful communication such as pointing, gesturing and miming fail to appear.

With more damaged children speech does not appear, and children try to communicate through the language of their organs. In normal sensory development, children increasingly learn to teach the body through a developing *sense of life,* usually resulting in the experience of a sense of self, as well as the release of language and the polarisation of self-experience with the perception of another person as another ego.

Thus, the speech disturbances of autistic children and their use of language are closely linked to retarded perception of the other person as an ego. Speech remains only a limited expression of self, occurring as echolalia or, if further developed, as a warding off of demands from the environment. Around the third year, it is especially frustrating for the mother, or another person new to the child, that they cannot make themselves understood to the child through language.

Early disturbance in making eye contact already indicates later problems in communication through speech with autistic children. Therefore, monitoring eye contact always plays an important part in the early recognition of autistic children. According to our observation, obtained mostly from mothers, children either make no eye contact at all or eye contact decreases the more they grow into earthly conditions and demands. Looking is an intentional act in which we participate intensely with our ego. The other person must be able to endure this gaze, to place something against it, otherwise eye contact cannot be maintained.

Normal children learn to place the experience of their own bodily nature, gained through the four lower senses, against this as a foothold in the world that can be seen by others, i.e. from outside. The lower senses are touch, life, movement and balance.

You will have noticed how careful one has to be, when making eye contact with a baby in its cradle. You then also see immediately that the therapeutic enforcement of eye contact, as practised for many years by behaviourist therapists, constitutes an inhuman overpowering of children and their own initiatives. However, the more we assist children in forming their own body-experiences as experiences of self in the field of the lower senses, the more they will perceive the gaze of someone else as communication and respond to it.

From this understanding, many therapeutical activities have resulted in the early treatment of these children. However, I only wish to point out that normally early eye contact between mother and child, usually in the course of the first weeks of life, begins to extend to objects, so that an inter-humanly constituted world of objects develops. In autistic children, this development is disturbed early on. The establishment of this shared world is, however, the prerequisite for the use of language as a means of reference between people.

Towards the end of the third year problems related to the experience of self in the child, through saying 'I', usually become fully apparent. Autistic children often call themselves 'you', although they are not awake to the ego of the other person as 'you'.

Rudolf Steiner showed that the perception of another person as an ego, as well as the perception of their language and thoughts, constitutes a direct sensory experience to which children, after birth, become increasingly awake. Up to the third year, the perception of another's ego as 'you' is formative for the child's awakening ego-consciousness, which has consolidated itself through the experience of the non-ego of the world of objects.

Through child development, experiences within the various areas of sense perception are made on different levels of consciousness, and a mere polarisation of consciousness and unconsciousness does not suffice for the theory of sense maturation. The connection between fully perceiving the self in the body, the awakening towards the world of objects, and the highest wakefulness in perceiving someone else, must develop in a harmonious relationship, which entails a well-developed ability to communicate together with the arising of one's inner ego-consciousness. However, the displacement of perceptive consciousness constitutes a central problem in the diagnosis and therapy of autistic children, and does not exist in this general form in any other learning difficulty (see von Arnim in König 1978).

Autistic children's lack of awakening to the perception of their fellow men, their thoughts, speech and ego-being, represents perhaps the most serious trauma for the relationship between children and their human environment. When children only perceive sequences of sound instead of the meaning of words, or only see another person as a thing among things, one can understand what this means for the parents of these children, and also perhaps for therapists. They are not perceived as soul-spiritual beings. This is significant for parents, and especially for mothers of autistic children, since the development of communication is a reciprocal relationship in which children increasingly perceive the people nearest to them on earth, acknowledge them, and thereby also contribute to *their* development as parents. This is especially clear with the first child of a family. The people nearest to these children become part of the autistic situation, for example, when children use their mother as an object to fulfil their wishes. As the other person is not being perceived, he or she is manipulated as an object in the environment. This parental experience seems to be representative of early childhood autism. There is no statistically or clinically objective diagnosis without reference to mutual experiences of communication.

The early symptoms mentioned so far are only indicative of the autistic syndrome if they appear, firstly, in groups and, secondly, over a prolonged period, and increase according to the dynamics of development, usually towards the third year in cases where early therapy did not take place. Many of the disturbances described, if they occur temporarily or in isolation, can point to critical phases of development in a normal child.

The paediatrician, when first confronted with autistic symptoms, must also consider comparative diagnoses of other developmental

215

disturbances that can occur in the first three years of life, from aetiologies which can cause autistic reactions. Here, one must take into consideration prenatal or perinatal brain damage, as well as the rather symptomless varieties of encephalitis that can occur in the first three years of life. One should be aware of the barely noticeable changes that may occur after smallpox inoculations, and that show autistic symptoms. Further attention should be paid to early symptoms of deafness, when speech does not develop after the babbling phase. Fundamental disturbances of visual perception, and in hearing and speech, should also be considered. These latter symptoms can only be eliminated over longer periods of observation and with repeated investigations. Moreover, autistic reactions can also appear as a result of prolonged hospitalisation or neglect. These can usually be overcome through a change of environment or therapy, but not always.

Early childhood neuroses, with delayed ego-maturation, which becomes apparent around the third year, can also show symptoms of an autistic reaction.

The 'autistic psychopathy' described by Asperger, usually with regard to early symptoms, shows a different course. The primary perceptive ability of a common world-of-action remains, and speech formation is mostly undisturbed. However, children shut themselves off in a world of their own, show intellectual abstract precociousness and flat soul-less forms of movement, often with a delayed development of the total psycho-motor co-ordination. As a rule this pattern only appears clearly around or after the third year, and according to generally available information, relates mostly to boys.

However, isolated symptoms before three years of age should not be seen as a primary declaration of the possible presence of childhood autism. Therefore, for the purpose of diagnosis and necessary therapy, several examinations and, whenever possible, prolonged observation and repeated conversations with parents over a longer period of time are necessary. Insufficient diagnostic clarification and early advice to parents, the absence of therapeutic attitudes directed to the development of imitation, and above all, early efforts at conditioning, can quickly lead to autistic situations between child and parents.

This then leads also to the increasing social isolation of the parents and, related to this, wrong attitudes towards the child. Consequently, the already problematic inter-human dynamic can be negatively influenced, often for a long time.

Contrary to Bettelheim's conception, with the children we have observed and treated over the last thirty years, there seems to be no direct parental cause of early childhood autism. We must, however, accept that considering the rhythmical relationship that exists from the start with their child, the parents find themselves in a situation where the child's disturbed actions and perceptions prevent the creation of a mutually accepted world. This situation often causes them to despair in their own role as parents, as they are increasingly forced to adopt a pedagogical attitude that often demands too much from the child. The earlier and the more intensively mere behavioural measures are offered to parents, the more medical doctors and therapists may themselves become part of the fundamental problem of communication in the framework of the family. This situation, therefore, requires more intensive initial work with the parents, which is necessary in the family situation where, especially if the autistic child is the first child, the relationship between the parents is often difficult. The father can withdraw after the birth of an autistic child, leaving the mother alone with the child. In this situation continuing advice and help are therapeutically necessary.

Through their disturbed perception, autistic children often become the mirror of their parents' behaviour and habits of relating. Normal children actively absorb these impressions, whereas in autistic children there is already a failure of imitation or a weakness of incorporation. The sooner after birth the child's autistic symptoms begin to show, the more fundamentally the developmental steps of the first three years appear to be disturbed. Early diagnosis and courses of therapy are therefore of decisive importance, and, above all, support for the people nearest to the child must be provided.

The child's weakness of incorporation is not genetically determined and in-born, but nevertheless it is in a certain sense *native* to the family situation. In the mothers of autistic children, quite frequently we find a relatively strong verbal-intellectual activity as part of their lifestyle and relationships. However, the lifestyle of the father, in our experience, is often marked through professional, or extra-professional special interest in his achievements, which is sometimes fanatically pursued. These parental attitudes are certainly not direct causes but often add to the picture of the family group. In the course of therapy with autistic children it is therefore suggested that the parents' habits of their inner and outer way of life are changed, so that they may become helpful partners in the destiny of their child. With regard to the problems of autistic children, the therapist is also continually called upon to be ready to give up certain habits, which in dealing with a normally developing child remain inconspicuous, since the child can cope actively and in a transforming way with them. However, the inability of autistic children to transform earthly experiences, in contrast to other learning difficulties, is especially pertinent to autism. Perceptions cannot unfold themselves in the dimension of time; they cannot be incorporated into the child's biography.

So, the need for intensive work with the parents is clear. This is usually prolonged, and takes a positive course when the initially isolated parents discover the curative educator to be actively participating in their situation.

I have tried to give some points of view of the curative educational diagnosis, based on spiritual science, for the early recognition of these children. From this, corresponding therapeutical beginnings can be made, aimed at solving the autistic isolation of child and family, and avoiding continuing damage through any inappropriate behaviour of children and their parents.

Part Two

People living with autistic children must realise as soon as possible that the symptoms – such as contact disturbances with other people, stereotypical behaviour and fixations – are not the illness itself, but desperate efforts to survive in a stressful, chaotic world of sense perceptions and relationships. In this effort, children's perceptual world, as well as their world of activity, becomes considerably narrower than it is for normally developing children. Through this situation the original expectations of parents are also deeply and lastingly disappointed.

A situation arises when the family's rhythms of life are so enduringly disturbed through a child's behaviour that the child's relationship with the family is reduced to mutual outer dependence and, finally, each only reacting to the other. Increasingly parents' ability to gain insight into ways in which they might help their child is lost. As a result, autistic children are often either challenged too much or too little.

Adopting a number of basic therapeutic attitudes can resolve this kind of situation, while involving a considerable and lasting adaptation of family habits. This appears to us to be the essential first step in therapeutic understanding before any special therapy exercises are implemented.

Basic therapeutic attitudes

1. Autistic children are not just handicapped or badly adjusted – they are injured by a world that is foreign to them. Their symptoms are efforts to find their way in this world within the specific limitations of their ability to relate.

2. Autistic children have a long way to go. Rapid results of adjustment may initially make family life easier. In the long run – and parents must learn to be prepared for this – what matters is the independence children achieve in their relationship with the world, also when this relationship seems different from what we are used to.

3. Nobody can manage the problems of these children alone. Therefore, as parents, look quickly for advice and assistance from other experienced parents, medical doctors and therapists.

4. It is not your personal fault that your child is autistic. As long as you think so you will demand too much from your child because you believe that you have to compensate for something.

219

5. Rather, create for yourself an attitude directed towards the real being of your child that lies behind the symptoms, and which wants to become healthy. Cultivate this attitude at all times, even when you are not with your child. It is an injustice to children if you only direct your attention to the symptoms of their behaviour.

6. As parents, discuss your experiences and observations together, so that you can find a common attitude. This will help your child, as otherwise one parent is often overstretched and the other not sufficiently engaged.

7. Autistic children have the inclination to reduce relationships of soul to relationships with objects. Perhaps your child sometimes treats you like an object.

8. Try to look for the true soul-spiritual being of your child behind the symptoms: a being that cannot grasp, or sufficiently penetrate, the physical body as an organ of perception and cognition.

9. Your child has the inclination to replace relationships with the living world of people with a fascination for gadgets, especially those of a technical kind. Strictly limit the use of tapes, television, computers, technical-didactic toys, etc.

10. What children need above all is access to simple human activities in which they can slowly learn to participate; for example, washing-up, laying the table, folding linen, looking after a flower etc.

11. Be critical in the matter of fixed programmes of education and therapy. You should act only after having acquired new therapeutic attitudes towards your child.

12. Above all, you need to employ compassion and loving observation when deciding what you can and cannot demand from your child. As parents you must agree on this, and what happens is ultimately dependent on your mutual understanding of your child. Try therefore, through your observations, to distract the child from an

expected act that is socially disturbing or self-destructive before you say no. Autistic children can be disturbing but they do not want to be so.

13. Plan your day in such a manner that at certain times you can devote yourselves entirely to your child. He needs a reliable rhythm and time when you fully turn to him. At first do simple things with your child, for example, guide his hand when he puts forks on the table or when he turns on a tap. Go on doing this until he can do some of these things on his own and/or imitates you.

14. Try, in the rhythm of your special times together, to stimulate reciprocal activity. Do not confront your child to begin with, but at first remain behind him, then next to him and then, finally, opposite him. Play reciprocal games, such as building bricks, saying rhythmically, 'I put a brick down, you put a brick down,' and apart from this, do not talk too much. With such simple games it is not a matter of construction, but of communication. Do not force any eye contact. That will come of its own accord to the extent that the child discovers you as a partner in a joint activity.

15. Do not talk too much or too little with children. Aim always for an increase in their perception of speaking. Speak simply and with gestures. Avoid intellectual language with a strong reflective element, as this is at first only noise to children.

16. Plan well what you wish to demand from your child as regards language. Do not expect the child to always immediately repeat what you say. In an appropriate situation say a word to the child and do this repeatedly and regularly, even for days and weeks, without always demanding that they repeat it. Learn to wait without becoming inert.

17. Refer everything you say to your child's ordinary surroundings. Try to increase the child's understanding

of simple sentences that express a request, rather than merely the imitation of single words. For example, 'Fetch that ball for me.'

18. Do not correct all the time. At first, allow your child to pass the sausages when they are asked to pass the butter. Initially, relate speech to actions, and later to instructions and objects. Avoid using words and pictures together. Children may perhaps manage to show the correct card for a word, but they do not know what is depicted. Children must first learn to live with the words in the actual world before the picture world is opened to them. This transition often occurs suddenly and unexpectedly, at first in only a few isolated situations.

19. Autistic children learn a lot in situations in which they are not confronted. You should take this into account. Autistic children notice more than you might at first assume. Speak softly, and not always from the front but also from behind, for autistic children are not yet self-assured when confronted by someone. In such situations children will do or say all kinds of things in order to be left in peace.

20. Do not talk about children in their presence.

21. Do support every spontaneous meaningful thing children do, through joining in or imitating them in confirmation.

22. Try to observe the rhythms of your child's life: the rhythms of sleeping and waking, eating and excretion. These rhythms are always disturbed, and as a result, the child does not appear to be socially adjusted. Try to alter these rhythms slowly to a reliable rhythm, by at first using strictly determined times. In some cases this can take months.

23. Autistic children also need other children, to whom they often appear less strange and distressing than

to adults. Depending on experience, you must decide between the fourth and seventh year of age whether your child will be educated at home, in a day kindergarten, in another therapeutic setting, or in a residential therapeutic centre outside the family. By this time you will have most of the experience needed to make such a decision. Autistic children do best among other children who are not all autistic. There is no scientifically valid theory of any kind which relieves you of this decision.

24. It is always important to see your child as an individual, and today there are enough experienced people who can advise you. Of course, these people occasionally have different ideas about what may be right in the situation. In any case, what is decided should specifically relate to your child, and not merely follow predetermined theories and models.

Aspects of schooling

1. Because of the autistic disturbance it is not easy to decide on the right kind of schooling for each child. The usual methods of testing do not provide sufficient criteria.

2. Therefore it is necessary to approach the total picture each autistic child presents with regard to:
   a. ability to meet others,
   b. perceptual areas available to them or in need of development,
   c. their independence relating to impulses of will,
   d. their ability to express themselves in gestures, play and language,
   e. their ability with regard to visual memory and other essential symbolic activities, such as perception of language.

3. From this it follows that only through prolonged

observation in a relevant class situation can specific ways be found to approach each autistic child.

4. A special factor here is how deeply established any pathological forms of reaction against the environment are, which would prevent the child's openness to learning.

5. Formal programmes of learning must therefore always be tested in relation to the personality of the child.

6. It is necessary, before school age, to establish whether the autistic behaviour of your child has any single determining cause, for instance, hearing damage, specific disturbances of language understanding or speech, or brain damage following an infection or encephalitis.

7. The extent of what can be asked of the child, and the kind of educational method and therapy, are dependent on such diagnostic clarifications, and you should get advice from an experienced child psychiatrist.

8. Autistic children have, in most cases, multiple-sensory difficulties, in that they are not able to integrate new sensory impressions in a meaningful way. This is especially apparent when one has the opportunity to live for years with autistic children. Autistic children need very small classes for schooling and some single one-to-one lessons, especially at first. These individual sessions cannot be limited to the area of school learning, but must also extend to special curative educational, therapeutic measures. However, the aim must always be that they become more and more able to integrate into the class group.

9. According to our experience, autistic children also need the presence of children with other learning difficulties within a class context (Feuser 1980).

10. Autistic children often show special abilities, such as a pronounced local memory, manual-technical skills and other intellectual semi-talents. This often leads

to the one-sided advancement of these talents. In the area of school, however, the aim is to work towards a harmonious, all-round development – in particular the educational-therapeutic cultivation of artistic and manual craft activities.

11. Above all, we should be aware that autistic children, during the course of their school time, and especially at the beginning of the third seven-year period (around fourteen years of age), go through considerable crises, but that even in these circumstances the ability to learn remains for a long time. However the initial autistic symptoms may change considerably over the course of the school years. Often stereotypical movements and fixations become less obvious and, as they grow older, children become more open to social relationships with other adults and children. The older autistic children become, the more they want to grow beyond their initial autistic situation or environment. For this, they need other children and adults as well as those in their own family.

12. It is especially important for autistic children – if it has not been prevented by earlier wrong approaches – that the ability to learn can continue for a long time, and therefore school and therapy should go on until the age of 21. This is a matter of fostering the disturbed earth-maturation of the ego. Autistic young people acquire identity especially through the acknowledged contribution they can make in practical activities, their experience of success and social recognition given to them by others.

13. Autistic children are autistic because they are culturally and socially isolated, through the fact that they cannot initially manage to make the world of their perceptions meaningful. The support of a therapeutic community of teachers, therapists and parents, and ultimately of

225

society in general is necessary to overcome this isolating environment. Therefore in the education of autistic children, the most important aim should be to enable these children to live as people, as freely as possible, albeit with difficulties, with other people in community.

13. The Topsy-Turvy World: An Anthroposophic Understanding of Autism in Early Childhood

From a privately published manuscript, 'Die verstellte Welt – Zum geisteswissenschaftlichen Verständnis des frühkindlichen Autismus', 1970.

Since autism in early childhood was first described by Leo Kanner and his collaborators in 1943 as a disorder of the affective contact with the environment, a great number of physicians, psychologists, therapists and curative educators have tried to come closer to an understanding of this disorder. In 1960, Karl König summed up the findings at that time in two lectures, and he made the first step towards a spiritual-scientific penetration of the phenenomenon. He especially pointed to the inability of these children to imitate. The stages of imitation that unfold and differentiate during the first seven years of life include children's ability to interiorise their human environment and thereby to make it their own.

This phenomenon of human development and learning, which is often not sufficiently acknowledged, signifies the early stage of inter-human relationships and recognition. As increasingly demonstrated by a multitude of observations during the last years, autistic children show a profound disorder, which is manifested quite early in life, on the level of relationships with the world. The most essential manifestations are summed up as follows:

1. The relationship with other human beings is disturbed or lacking altogether. Children do not react to the

speech or gesture of other people; they avoid their gaze
and sometimes also touch.

2. Autistic children do not experience things within
   a human space of reference, but in relation to their
   position in geometric space (situation, position, relation,
   form), and strive towards uniformity of spatial object
   arrangements and sequences in time.

3. If autistic children can speak, they use words as if they
   were things, in a way that does not include meaning or
   relationship to the environment. The personal pronouns
   'I' and 'you' are often exchanged. With regard to these
   linguistic connections, G. Bosch (1962) published an
   important study based on phenomenological points
   of view (see also Rutter 1978; Schopler 1978; Kehrer
   1978).

Here, then, the basic phenomena are mapped out which, since
Kanner's descriptions, have been verified by almost all authors, and
which in all their many variations show the disturbed relationships of
autistic children to their surroundings and contemporaries. When we
meet autistic children we have to be clear that their world is not just
deficient to ours, but see that they create a private world in which they
can live, even though this world appears narrowed down to us and, to
begin with, unapproachable.

The spiritual-scientific knowledge of the senses, described by
Rudolf Steiner (1981), differentiates different fields of perceptions,
which results in a realm of higher, middle and lower (or body) senses.

These differentiations have proved particularly fruitful for
understanding autistic children, but also for approaching other
developmental disorders. I will often refer back to the spiritual-scientific
understanding of the senses in the course of these contemplations
(Steiner 1980; Lauer 1977).

Sensory experience and the development of consciousness

Soon after birth, autistic children show behaviour which is often overlooked and which points to their inability to grasp their inter-human environment. There is no response to maternal care. In the gaze, in smiling, in the corresponding movement of the arms when mothers lift children from the cradle, every original contact seems to be lacking that would otherwise make up the richness of the early mother-child relationship. Mothers who relate instinctively to their child as a responding soul-being, sense this disorder in pre-verbal relationship. However, mothers who concentrate chiefly on the bodily needs of their child often overlook this deficiency, and only notice it later between the second and third years of life when the child does not communicate through gesture or language. These occurrences, which are fundamental to the mother-child relationship, have been the subject of many valuable observations and investigations which all concur in recognising the significance of early experiences of environment for the entire development of the emotional and recognitional functions.

What happens during the first months of life belongs to the recurring mystery of archetypal human encounter, by which the ego of the child actively integrates into the surrounding human world and culture and, by way of imitation, makes this world the child's own: part of his body. The growing child first relates to objects – a chair, a spoon – because the mother or care giver and the child share attention in this object. Later the child can independently name the object, a spoon, and use it for communication. Among the many phenomena that show children's participation with their human environment, it is through smiling that what really matters can best be shown.

Through children smiling on meeting their mothers, a bodily participation with the environment comes to expression, or, through the higher senses the soul-attitude of the mother is experienced. More precisely, the newborn child primarily perceives the given intentions of the mother, still far removed from the ability to objectify the outer bodily form of the mother. This encounter finds a response in the plasticity of the body, which appears in the expression of smiling.

229

As children experience themselves in their mothers, so mothers experience themselves in the responding smiles of their children.

We notice here one of the many encounters of early childhood, which we can describe as the formative circle of mutual human acknowledgment which, as we will see, is similar to the instinctive behaviour of animals, and yet is fundamentally different. Child and mother awaken to themselves, and thereby construct a mutual environment in the process of human relationships. Revealed in this process is a stage of imitation first described by Rudolf Steiner, the primary happening of which lies in the sensory activity of the child meeting the empathy of the mother. Basic to this is an active process of seeking and finding in the child, which E.H. Erikson simply and truthfully called hope, which:

> ...grows out of the unbroken early trust and mutuality
> and produces a feeling of fitting into the personal and
> cultural environment ... As a consequence this hope is
> always filled again through all those rituals and ritualising
> which are engaged against the feeling of forsakenness and
> hopelessness and, instead of this, promise throughout life
> a mutual recognition face to face until we recognise that
> we are recognised. (Erikson 1968)

Child psychology has only in the last twenty years started to recognise and understand the active achievement of children in integrating themselves, or participating, in the mutual and also personal world, and has thereby focused on the intentionality of the soul-spiritual centre of children's being. In a treatise on the essential aspects of autism in early childhood, J. Lutz has pointed to ego-activity and its weakness in autistic behaviour, by clearly showing it as the:

> ...individual kernel of the human being ... Through the
> activity of this kernel the human being grasps the world,
> becomes conscious of himself in the world, and senses his
> connection with spiritual powers. (Lutz, 1968)

230

The forms of early inter-human encounter, from the morning greeting by the mother to the moment she says goodnight, which Erikson called ritualising, help integration into the shared environment, including tuning-in with the child's bodily experiences in this world. There is an interaction between the experiences of the surrounding world and the bodily experiences of the child, in thirst, hunger, positions and movements, and also tension within organs. Small children perceive all of these phenomena with the lower senses more intensively than later on and, every time, these expressions of the children's perceptions are met with the tuned-in behaviour of the mother as a response.

In these early stages, children do not yet experience their bodies as their own. They are, to begin with, bound up with the presence of the mother, and the bodily functions, which are not yet organised instinctively, still require a long time of body and soul care by the mother. At stake are time-giving inter-human rhythms which are, from the outset, not grasped by autistic children. Therefore, these children are thrown back on to their own bodily existence, which has not yet achieved an organised self-recognition, quite early.

In normal development, the experience of the child's own body as a personal world, and the perception of other human beings as independent people, occurs through the active grasping and taking hold of the world of things. This begins in the first year of life as a process leading to the objectifying of the world, and signifies a gradual alienation from the closed mother-child relationship. The archetypal reciprocity of encounter and the early connection of body experience and environment experience, as described above, undergoes a change. The world of things, of objects, transmitted by the senses of seeing, hearing, smelling and tasting, appears increasingly dominant in the child's consciousness, and consolidates the self-consciousness of the child *vis-à-vis* the world. The grasping and seeing of the world of things in their surroundings signifies a crossing point in child development. They experience their body as an object among objects, and begin to construct their own world over and against their surroundings, and this remains then unmistakenly their own for all their life on

231

earth. Normally developing children begin to be able to experience, 'having a body and at the same time being a body' (see von Arnim in König 1966). Simultaneously with increased objectifying, perception of the surroundings begins to change from its original joint action to a pictorial recognition. The imitating joint action in the human world remains up to the seventh year. In this the ego seizes itself as a self *vis-à-vis* its surroundings. Rudolf Steiner described in detail this process of increasing individualisation through increasing pictorial conceptions in the first year of life. Jean Piaget described in countless observations the change from the world of imitation to the world of images (Piaget 1962).

The non-achievement of objectifying in autistic children makes the world of objects appear as belonging to their own bodies. The objects do not assume the character of a challenge to deal with actively; they do not become subjects of verbal references, nor do they engage the conceptual-pictorial activity of thinking. One can describe the gravity of this disorder as a limitation of the space of freedom, which normally, and in contrast to animals, consists in the manifold availability of the world of objects for action and play, for talking about them with somebody, and for forming mental images and memories.

Following the spiritual-scientific investigations of Rudolf Steiner (1970), we have to assume that the lack of objectifying of the world has its roots in the disability of autistic children to arrive at a conceptual judgment of perception in relation to the reality of the world of objects. This would normally express itself in consciousness as an acknowledgment that something *is*, relatively independent of myself, and yet in relation to myself and to other people as a common world reality. The fact that the classical natural scientific trend of thought equates the concept of reality with matter shows that science has omitted to recognise this concept as a perceptual judgment. This has thereby caused the component of objectifying in child development to be overlooked, which we then meet in autistic children as a disorder.

The role of the lower senses

In living with autistic children, it is clear that they do not discover the sphere of co-existence. Rarely is the gaze of such children directed at another human being, their movements remain unrelated to the intentions of other people in gesture or expression, and things of common use are not integrated into the same human space of relations and meaning; they are not objectified. We gain the impression that autistic children, because of this primary disability, do not discover the world of images and pictorial memories, and cannot freely dispose of these within their soul. Instead, biographically irrelevant stereotypic forms of memory arise, often bound to space and locality.

The process of individualisation, towards the seventh year of life, is only partially achieved, and therefore the bodily gestalt, facial expressions and movement patterns remain almost unchanged up to the seventh year. Movement patterns and gestalt achieve some personal limited dynamic of habit, which consist in the manipulation of objects, and take place in space apart from human encounter.

For autistic children things gain significance in space according to their position, size and form. Children aim to create compulsively, through rites and numbers, a closed space that renders them some security. This is quite different from the certainty of self-assuredness brought about through recognised and remembered images, or through verbally transmitted contents which mediate the double experience of time, as past or as an opportunity for freely planning the future.

We can understand this closed space as one in the present; it is unhistoric and abstract, cut off from the fullness of possible human changes, especially from any involvement with, or openness to, other people. It becomes a dead space without development. Autistic children are therefore adjusted to the spatial arrangements of things. They try to establish a closed space that is perfect in the arrangement of things, simulating security, yet excluding inter-human intentions and meanings. One of our children continuously places toy bricks in straight lines or circles, which is typical of this behaviour. At mealtimes, the moment a child at another table hands her plate to her group mother, the autistic child jumps up and places his plate in front of her; the order of the circle has been disturbed, an opening has appeared, and the boy rushes to repair the circle with his own plate.

Any changes and additions, and sometimes even the intentional gaze of another person, can be experienced with horror and panic, as disturbances of this ordered environment. G. Bosch discussed the question of intersubjective objectification, which means that a thing can be seen differently through the eyes of another person. Bosch concludes correctly that autistic children mainly show interests that do not require extensive objectification within a common world, or only to a small degree.

With autistic children we also experience other characteristic ways of dealing with things. Synonymous with the concept of fixing or determining a position in space, there seems to be a special kind of sensory experience which produces an objectifying along the lines of classical physics. This reduces the world to identities of number and measure. Such data in space, that is, pseudo-facts, are taken as the starting point, which then excludes the element of reality. Autistic children deal similarly with the spoken word, which is reduced to a verbalisation independent of any context, which is then applied in all circumstances.

With this concept of fixing, it should be made clear that this is a specific divergent structuring of the world of perceptions. We further notice that their manipulation of things, as well as their own body movements, shows a rhythm which, as in mechanisms, works as a closed system. The rhythmic movements of their own body-object can extend without transition to: the manipulation of light switches or taps; the compulsory opening and closing of doors; the continuous fitting together of shapes, such as in jigsaw puzzles; the piecing together and taking apart of mechanical, and often very complicated, items; repetitions of tunes; or the picking up again of the same activity, in which the repetition might take minutes or months. The attention of these children seems drawn into a magic circle of the relationships of size, number and weight, which they seek to make real.

In this phenomenon, too, we find the important rhythm of

temporal-historic, inter-human relationships and ritualisations, games with objects, and the life rhythm of sleeping and waking turned into something spatial. A kind of limited rhythm of self, which is non-pictorial and lacking history, replaces and annuls interpersonal communication. Generally, rhythmic happenings in the normal development of early childhood are shown as the phenomenon of encounter: in glancing and turning away, in grasping and letting loose, in taking possession of and yielding an object, and many other rhythmically bound and repetitive achievements. However, the reduction of the rhythmic circumference leads, on the one hand, to movement and action stereotypes, and on the other hand, to a compulsory fixation in sensory experiences and to the obsessive need to repeat. Later, in the development of these children, these repetitions become habitual. The discovery of such disturbances of rhythm seems important, and significant therapeutic consequences have followed with regard to shaping life-rhythms for these children.

A third phenomenon, which we observe time and again, refers to relationships of balance. One of our children went through a phase in which he placed all kinds of objects along the edge of a table just preventing them from falling down, or he placed toy bricks on top of each other to a height no other child could have achieved.

We have also discovered the preference of these children for symmetry. One of our children, for many days, took all the shoes out of the wardrobe and separated the left ones from the right ones; he put the right shoes on one side of the passage and the left shoes on the other side. The toes were placed exactly opposite each other. Such symmetrical arrangements can also be found in the placing of toy bricks or crayons in colour or mirror patterns. Another child, when asked to push in a drawer, pulled out all the other drawers to exactly the same extent, so that they agreed mathematically. In this instance, an obsessive spatial-geometric arrangement was satisfied by sacrificing the functional use of a drawer, i.e. for pulling out or pushing in.

Finally, we should mention another behaviour that supplies further hints as to the kind of world an autistic child constructs, which is linked with the sense of touch. Frequently we see autistic children observe objects, such as a chair, from all sides. With their gaze they follow the structure of the chair exactly, along the back, around the seat; they turn the chair round, creep under it, as if they wanted to touch all its spatial dimensions – angles, lines, whether straight, round or diagonal – with their eyes. Watching such a child intensively, one can experience how the sensory activity of seeing does what is otherwise done by the sense of touch. The sense of touch, however, only informs us of the boundary of our own body. Autistic children therefore miss out the image-experience and meaning of an object, and only recognise the spatial aspect in an autonomous, closed space.

When we consider these dimensions of the autistic world, we can conclude that this world is limited to the experience of the lower senses – the senses of balance, own movement, life and touch. Throughout the first seven years of normal child development, these four senses provide the perception of our own body as self-world, which comes into relationship with the world of things and the human environment. They thereby allow the self to become aware, as ego, within its bodily existence and within a differentiated world. However, in autistic children, the self-world of the body is not individualised, but instead is fused unhealthily with their perceptions of the environment. Autistic children distort the experience of their own body as an intact self-experience, as well as their encounter with the environment. They are imprisoned in the world of the lower senses, which invades the field of the middle senses – the senses for perceiving the environment – and does not allow these to unfold. Edmund Husserl maintains that experiences gained by solipsistic means are irreconcilable with experiences made by others. [*Solipsism*: from the Latin *solus* (alone) and *ipse* (self). Originally used as a term for practical egoism, *solipsism* was used in the late nineteenth century from the theoretical view that only I and my experiences exist.] He pointed out that, 'Free from the need of confirmation through the other person and independent from inter-subjective objectification, are only such experiences which are objectified by logic-mathematical laws.'

According to Husserl, only things based on measurement, number and weight justify themselves; that is, all logically, mathematically confirmed constitutions carry their objectification within themselves, and are independent of place, time and human fellowship (Bosch 1962).

In comparing this with the behaviour of autistic children, the following should be considered. The ability to think in abstract terms is usually only achieved at the end of the second seven-year period of development, and is based on, and maintained by, a confirmed experience of the environment. This ability is not primarily present in the field of sensory perception, but rests on the secondary formation of concepts based on the matured lower senses: namely the senses of life, movement, balance and touch. In autistic children, however, these secondary forms of thinking become the content of primary world-structuring by means of the lower senses. Autistic children actually seem to awaken too early with regard to the environment, and are then unable to make the step into the world of images and inter-human relationships.

Rudolf Steiner was the first person to indicate the connection between our body perception given through the lower senses and mathematical-geometrical thinking. He described at length how geometrical activity, the rhythms of number sequences, the laws of conclusion and logical judgment in relation to the laws of space in general have evolved from experiences made through the four lower senses, which then appear as laws in the thinking consciousness. In contrast, however, the perceptions of the lower senses remain largely unconscious. Indeed they actually become unconscious during the first year of life, in order to give the senses of sight, taste, smell and temperature the opportunity to construct the outer world and, in conjunction with the higher senses, to also construct the social world with others.

We may then assume that autistic children become too awake in the lower senses, whose primarily spatial qualities of recognition are given scope among the environmental senses, especially in seeing. Thereby the environment becomes a one-sided spatial world which cannot be communicated unless first turned into secondary mathematical or geometric concepts and conceptions.

A six-and-a-half-year-old autistic girl impressively demonstrated her transition from a closed self-world towards the mutual co-existent world. At the age of four, she still showed all the signs of a severe autistic contact disturbance, but she slowly learned to enter the world of images and speech. These tender relationships to the co-existent world are still insufficiently developed, and she still always makes her spatial security arrangements. For example, she arranges the beads in different rows on the abacus: she calls the uppermost and longest father, the tallest in the family; followed by granny in a slightly shorter row; then mother in the next row; followed by her older sister; then herself and little brother. The human relationships here find expression according to size, which have, however, already taken on symbolical character representing the co-existent world. Here, too, disturbances appear in the experience of time; that is, the age differences among the members of the family shown as spatial constructions.

Our observations serve to show that autistic children fashion a closed spatial world for themselves, to which the child alone belongs and which alone promises security. This world represents a self-world that cannot be shared. This world is derived from the logical, mathematical form of thinking, underpinning a counting and calculating modern science, which today manifests itself increasingly as a determining factor in culture in the realm of technology. The intention behind it is perfection: a closed system, with the exclusion of any interference, of inter-subjective spaces of relationships; a world that functions and is tied, with the presumed and illusory expectation of security and complete control. It appears the more children with autism can create sameness in their environment, the more secure they can feel. They would like to have eternal sameness, without human beings disturbing their safe place. In our culture we know many such environments; think about a factory, where machines produce cars without human intervention. The appearance of autistic children in our present civilisation therefore seems to mirror the culture, stemming from the nineteenth century and reaching into our time, of a natural scientific technological worldview governed by logic and outer necessities.

Incomplete incarnation

Everyone who seeks lively contact with autistic children asks the question: what makes these children live in a world closed to others, and how can we learn to understand the origin of their behaviour?

This question becomes ever more urgent, and the answers to date are contradictory and insufficient. At the present stage most of the presented theories attempting to recognise the causes cannot be upheld. This disorder is neither genetically nor biologically inherited, nor, in the cases of most of the children, can brain-organic disturbances be proved. More importantly, it is generally accepted that culturally and socially-determined characteristics of the parents, and related aspects of their mismanagement, while revealing a situation of destiny, cannot be the primary cause of it. Kanner and Eisenberg pointed to a frequent, yet not always present, parental pattern of behavior, which they characterised as, 'the mechanising of human relationships' or the 'unconditional surrender to the principles of perfectionism'.

Such parents seem to take the 'obsessional sticking to rules and prescriptions' as a 'substitute for joy in life ... Mother and child live in bodily proximity and yet move in different spheres' (Fischer 1965).

We have begun to assume that these children forgo the normal adjustment to the human, cultural, co-existing world. Not only do parents receive their child but, and spiritual-science points to this, the newborn child is from the beginning actively engaged and seeks human connections in an intentionality which originated prenatally. The failure which seems particularly important with autistic children is the lack of an intentional attitude. After birth, children remember the prenatal archetype of their human environment and can open up to it. Rudolf Steiner exemplifies this using to the phenomenon of imitation:

> The child only continues, when entering through birth
> into physical existence, what he has experienced in the
> spiritual world before conception. As a human being
> one lives then within the beings of a higher order, and
> one does all the things which emanate as impulses from

239

the beings of this higher order. One is then to a much
higher degree an imitator, because one is at-one with
those beings whom one imitates. Then one is placed
outside into the physical world. This is, so to say, the
first birth, and one continues the habit to be at one with
one's surrounding. This habit embraces the beings who,
as human beings, appear in the surrounding and whom
one imitates. It is a much greater blessing for the child, the
more he need not live in his own soul, but the more he
can live in the soul of the environment, in the soul of his
fellow human beings. (Steiner 1997)

This symbiosis can go wrong when the child forgets the real
intentions of imitating this living together. Subsequently the world of
conceptual images, arising after the first objectification, may partially
succeed but will also suffer mishap. These conceptual images derive
from prenatal formative forces and are not only a reflection of a
physical-sensory, thought-out world (Steiner 1996).

We can then consider this primary failure in relation to the world of
autistic children, which is not composed of fellow human relationships
of confidence, hope and security, or constructed as a cultural-historic
world. Instead children become unhealthily awake in the field of earth
forces, which normal children dimly experience through the lower
senses. This field, too, is one of destiny, and is initially not conscious
to children but influences their development. Normal children realise
their destiny through action and trust, and through encountering a
co-existent world (Poppelbaum 1959). Autistic children, however, fail
to accept the world of destiny of their own doings and actions, which
normal children do through guidance of spiritual powers, and instead
construct a closed, spatially-bound world granting them pseudo-
security. Their destiny cannot unfold because they rigidify within
the wakefulness of their lower senses, in relation to measure, number
and weight, what should only be undertaken as tasks later on in the
secondary life stage of free formation of concepts.

These children therefore become awake in a reversal of consciousness of incarnation directions with regard to the sleeping intentions of destiny working in the life of will, and omit the wakeful consciousness of self within the sensory circumference of human fellowship.

H.E. Lauer, following the indications of Rudolf Steiner, has described how cosmic laws from prenatal life reveal themselves in the lower senses. In early childhood these experiences become bodily, and thereby also unconscious, in order to reappear later on as mathematical and geometric laws. Autistic children, instead of forgetting, seem to remember these systems of laws and to construct a self-world that falls prey to the laws of space. By failing to incarnate into human fellowship and relationships and forgetting themselves, but instead remembering and awakening in cosmic prenatal laws, autistic children omit to grasp their own body as bearer of action and destiny.

In order to become a self-conscious, active person, a dullness in the lower senses has to develop, and an awakening to the objects of the environment. In normal early childhood development, true self-motivated action and the distanciating from things only appears after the accomplishment of objectification. Then children experience themselves as acting, and realise that their body's manifestation in acting takes place within a co-existent world, which can see and experience them. This means that the body becomes an object among others, when the objectification is achieved during the second year of life (see Piaget).

Autistic children's lack of experience of the existence of their body, for themselves and others, is clear. We notice how vulnerable such children can be when, through a sudden confrontation, gaze or touch by another person, they feel exposed; this gives the impression that many of their behaviour patterns are geared not to be seen. To be seen is, however, an essential phenomenon of fellow-human relationships, by which the ego in its revelation through the body has to prove itself and becomes subject to correction. Individual children who reveal themselves in action recognise themselves not only in the dull perception of the body senses, but also through the gaze and relating attitudes of other people. In the early childhood relationship to the co-existent world, the environment plays a decisive role by the way in which it responds to the first revelations of child-like motivation. When we succeed in awakening even the smallest motivated action in autistic children, within an inter-human situation, an important step has been made along their own path of destiny, and for opening up their self-world, which is hemmed in by objects. In the first phase of therapy, autistic children often try for a long time to avoid another person's interest in their own actions. The growing tolerance of the child to be taken seriously, as a being acting in space, presents an important process in relationship forming. In his biographical-analytical monograph on autism, Bettelheim has been able to demonstrate just this process very convincingly (1967).

In conclusion, a path to an understanding of autism has been shown, through the insights of anthroposophy in early childhood development. The aim of this attempt is to render the curative educational encounter with autistic children in accordance with destiny; to deepen it, and foster a curative educational attitude which, in the long course of development of these children, opens up a life in a human world that is common to us all.

14. The Curative Educational School: Observations and Aims

Part One

Taken from a report to the first German Federal Council for Help for the Autistic Child, given in December 1972. It was revised and printed in the conference proceedings of the same council.

When we began to work with autistic children in the early fifties in Camphill schools in Scotland, under the leadership of Dr Karl König, we still called them, in accord with a widely used Anglo-Saxon concept, 'pre-psychotic children'. These pre-psychotic children formed a large group which, in treatment, care and education, we tried to distinguish from the so-called psychotics; that is, those with early childhood schizophrenia. Since then we have learned to observe and progress with these children through curative education. A great number of specific therapies and teaching methods have been developed, yet one cannot say that a model therapy or curriculum has evolved that would suit all such children. Nevertheless, since that time we have tried to admit children in our schools with early childhood autism, and to further them in every possible way.

From the beginning, we adopted the view that it is not necessarily the task of society or schools to educate these children according to fixed programmes. Rather we respect the reality that all children have a special destiny in this world, to which their parents also belong. We have also had the opportunity to follow the progress of a number of these children into young adulthood, each in their own particular life situation. They have learned, as adults, to live together with other people, though in a way specific to each of them, and perhaps without being able to understand or live in the real diversity of human life. The goals we set ourselves regarding curative education relate to three areas:

1. To make it possible for autistic children to gain the experience of self *vis-à-vis* the world.
2. To help children unfold some of their own initiatives, which become understandable and acceptable within a meaningful human field of interaction, in spite of fixed, stereotypical and sometimes obsessive patterns of behaviour.
3. To lead autistic children towards what is generally called 'symbolic understanding'. By this we mean the general comprehension of the significance of actions, of human expression and physiognomy, which healthy children develop during early childhood, and essentially before the acquisition of language.

Early childhood autism is recognised as a syndrome displaying disturbances in different dimensions such as thinking, feeling, speaking and acting. Therefore it is necessary to get to know these three areas more precisely.

Firstly, the so-called cognitive deficits of autistic children mean that they do not understand a word or action, and that they cannot grasp the time factor in changes within the environment of objects and things. Furthermore, they cannot relate an important life event to themselves, or can only perceive a fragment of such an event. All of these deficits have to be taken into account when considering the relationship of these children to their human environment.

The second area is the cognitive one that relates to human relationships in the true sense. We believe however that the term 'cognitive' is too narrow for this dimension as, especially in early childhood development, one cannot separate the realm of the sensory-cognitive from that of the feeling life of the child, which is often termed the 'emotional' or 'affective'. In practice, therefore, whether a therapy aims at the cognitive level or at the feeling life of the child is a superfluous question. In the therapeutic encounter with a young child, you cannot separate the therapeutic attitude from curative educational practice.

The third area of treatment is, according to our own estimate, the most important one. This relates to the enhancement of will, which means intentions, and the formation of the imaginative faculties and motives of the child, which also extend to the inter-human area of perception. We notice that many autistic children act particularly quickly when engaged in activities. This is especially evident in school, where they perform everything asked of them as if they want to get it behind them as quickly as possible, as if they have no time. Furthermore, autistic children show a pattern of behaviour that does not include other people in their field of activity. This situation is in the true sense of the word *autistic*, and it is difficult to change. Ultimately the action-behaviour of autistic children, which in classical descriptions is termed 'sameness', is significant. This concept signifies that autistic children are anxious to maintain the spatial arrangements in their surroundings and that they therefore resist any spatial change. We notice that this anxiety relates particularly to children's own activity. For example, if they are supposed to move from one room to another, they are likely to stop at the threshold, rock to and fro or make stereotypical movements, and not cross the threshold. We have experienced this in a variety of situations, where a child was meant to do something, yet felt unable and made a number of peculiar movements of a ritualistic kind instead. As a therapist, if one has the necessary flexibility, one will not only observe such behaviour but engage oneself, and often it is enough to take children by the hand and lead them across the threshold. This is usually successful if one's own intentionality is placed quietly and surely at the disposal of the child, and without causing arguments.

Doing something and moving oneself are not mere simple motor phenomena to be explained by neurology, but are human activities occurring in a mutual space of intentionality and meaning; one that

245

is, to begin with, closed to autistic children. Belonging to this space of meaning is essentially the permanent experience of one's own body as a reality. We believe that when autistic children are asked to do something but feel they can't, such as crossing the threshold from one room to another, they are frightened of being lost. Normally children overcome this anxiety by relating everything they do, including their own movements in space, to certain perceptions that they hold on to and with which they identify: primarily the experience of their own body. This seems to be disturbed in autistic children and they feel anxiety about losing themselves when they make a movement in action or speech.

This also appears to us to be the reason why autistic children, in daily life with their parents, fix on certain recurring habits of behaviour, expecting always the same reaction to the same actions. Therein lies the difficulty in handling autistic children. Not only do children demand the wrong self-assurance through the behaviour pattern of parents, but the parents generally expect normal and familiar reactions from children. As a result, a vicious circle can develop, which severely disturbs the family and tends to become obsessional, leaving no opportunity for free decisions. The exclusive behaviour of autistic children also makes it hard for parents to enter into, and participate in, the closed circle of their child's activities. This situation, which can generally be termed the 'autistic situation', occurs mostly between the third and seventh year of life, when it is most necessary to advise parents.

There are a number of schools whose policy is to promote intimate body contact between autistic children and their parents in early childhood. This bodily rhythm plays a decisive part in the earliest, natural contact between a mother and her child, and is seen as preceding linguistic-symbolic behaviour. With many autistic children, a disturbance appears soon after birth in the rhythm and soul interaction between mother and child. For example, they might not lift their arms when a parent tries to help them into their jacket, or not respond to a smile or when spoken to. These patterns reveal the basic lack of inter-human relationship.

246

In each case, parents should be considered carefully to see how much they are capable of contributing to a therapeutic process and seeing it through. In many cases parents cannot be productively involved at start of their child's educational process. They often find themselves trapped in a vicious circle of behaviour patterns, and it is helpful if the child, for a certain time, is away from home in order to break this circle and to allow everyone some respite from the autistic situation. In any event, every single case should, of course, be considered with reference to the situation of the parents and the parent-child relationship when deciding which particular therapeutic and educational course to follow. During a child's stay in a residential school, regular contact with and reports from co-workers give parents the opportunity to get to know their child anew.

From the beginning we have believed that autistic children should be cared for in special schools. However, time and again objections are raised, and care in a special school is deemed inappropriate because of the relatively high IQ evident in some of these children. Our experience shows, however, that it is important to realise that we are dealing with a syndrome, and that the emotional and will-disturbances, understood as intentionality, play a decisive role in the life of the child. The problem that arises relates to what kind of school is most beneficial for autistic children.

From the very start we decided not to found a school admitting only autistic children. We were guided by the fact that human life, especially in its unconscious dimension, is based on a wide range of encounters and experiences within the social field. For the conscious part of the human being it may appear differently, and a specialised training pro-gramme for autistic children may seem of importance. However, one should not underrate the subconscious factor of children's participa-tion in their environment. This is paramount for autistic children. After taking our lead from this, it became evident that within groups as well as in the class situation, children can help each other. Other children who do not show the same behaviour pattern, but are marked by their openness in dealing with the world, as is the case with Downs syndrome children, can especially help the autistic ones. They can break through the closed circle of autistic children, taking an autistic friend by the arm to go for a walk or look at something together; even doing something together that might not have been achieved by the group leader or teacher. The communality among children with learning difficulties is an important aspect of a school class or a group. The special blessing of such a therapeutic community, according to our experience, is shown particularly after the seventh year of life when normal children also seek contact with children of their own age.

If this proves successful, one might have the first clue to understanding why many autistic children become relatively normal between the ages of eight and nine, and manage to enter into an ordered human environment, whereas before that time they displayed considerable inter-human disorders. The world of early childhood and relationships starts to objectify, and children are able to have new experiences and encounters with new kinds of people. We should give this opportunity to autistic children.

We do not consider special schools only as academic institution, but as part of the framework of a therapeutic community where we also work with the children in curative educationally-oriented groups, and in home groups of five to six children. Therefore, specific therapeutic and curative educational approaches are integrated into our special school programme, together signified by the term, 'curative educational school'.

An autistic child joining a school class at the age of six or seven adjusts quite quickly, according to our experience, provided that some essentials of the learning process are taken into consideration. Autistic children gain more from lessons than they can show and it is possible, with the repetition of well-structured tasks, for children to truly assimilate the subject if sufficient time is granted. To this end it is important that the main subject lessons are presented in block periods, so that after three to four weeks children have taken in part of what has been offered. Any form of learning pressure is avoided.

From investigations concerning long- and short-term memory, it is clear that there is a great danger in training autistic children for particular academic successes, which are then reproduced in a stereotyped manner, since their long-term memory, which is also a biographical one, is only insufficiently or not at all developed. It is up to the teacher to avoid such a training process, otherwise children might be prevented from learning anything new. Autistic children place the highest demands on the therapeutic imagination and patience of the teacher.

Furthermore, a number of sensory exercises are included in the education of these children, designed specifically to enhance their own body perception through the so-called lower senses. These are the sense of balance, movement, life and touch (König 1986). For example, children can be encouraged to learn to draw shapes or letters with their finger in sand without using their eyes, and to recognise them by touching. Thereby a letter or word read by touching becomes real.

Movement exercises and movement games are especially valuable. In our schools a special form of movement, called eurythmy, is available. Using this approach one can present the word 'tree' to children in its sound formation, by first demonstrating the sequence of sounds in eurythmy movements, and then letting children repeat each letter. The first step is to make a word perceptible in its phonetic gestalt. When this has been achieved one can proceed to the symbolic meaning of the words.

In the realm of music we have introduced other exercises. A note is sounded on an instrument and the child is asked to sound the same tone in response. In this way small tone sequences or melodies arise. Especially during the early stages of this exercise interpersonal contact can be much improved.

At a later stage, we attempt play therapy by offering autistic pupils the opportunity to play with younger children, with dolls or other objects.

We know that autistic children when confronted with a jigsaw puzzle will quickly place the correct pieces without even looking at the picture. Here, too, it is apparent that other people are excluded from the child's field of action. However, in a therapeutic situation the therapist sits, to begin with, next to or behind the child, and only later opposite the child, and tries as much as possible to gain a reciprocal relationship; for example, by handing a brick to the child, who then hands it back to the therapist, so that gradually they build something *together*.

The therapeutic aim is to make it clear to the child: what I do, you can see; what I do, you can do; what you do, I can do; what you do, I can see. Such simple attitudes and therapeutic experiments, often in a very short time, unlock the closed play orbit of children and change it to togetherness in play. The best opportunities for this are before the age of seven.

We also engage children in warming therapy, founded on the observation that when autistic children have a raised temperature, they appear to be almost normal: stereotypical behaviour recedes, eye contact becomes clearer and, in such situations, one succeeds easily in playing with children; sometimes even speech disturbance is lessened. As a result, we administer carefully monitored hot baths, and it is surprising to see how children react to these in a relaxed way (Klimm 1965). Simultaneously there arises a noticeable openness to interpersonal contact, although to begin with this only lasts for a short time. Following this hyper-warming, the therapist plays and speaks with the child.

All these therapeutic measures are integrated with teaching and socialising in the group, within the setting of the curative educational school. With regard to the socialising process in general, we want to give autistic children the possibility of living within a human universe. However, autistic children, like normal children, become more distant from the world between the ninth and twelfth years of life. This distancing, which in autism already presented a pathological phenomenon in early childhood, is now more accepted and integrated by the child and others. It is noticeable that autistic children prefer to use any kind of medium in their dealing with the world rather than being confronted. Sometimes they learn more quickly to write with a pencil, some even with a typewriter, rather than speak. There are children who find their approach to speaking via spelling and reading. Normal steps of learning often come in the reverse, so that speaking is linked to reading. With older children especially, the therapeutic approach is directed at the person and not the symptoms, therefore also respecting and accepting a certain distance, through an enhanced paedagogic consciousness.

The destiny of autistic children maturing into adolescents varies considerably according to the individual. There are those who, after dramatic developments in early childhood, slowly grow into a reassured life situation and create an environment for themselves within which they can exist. These children clearly show what they want and, when one responds positively, they can maintain this habit, which however remains limited. If accepted, an important satisfaction is evident in the child. On the other hand there are also children who, in spite of all efforts, remain searching for their own identity, who are in a kind of limbo and never feel at home in this world. These children are the most difficult and they frequently develop symptoms similar to psychosis around their thirteenth, fourteenth and fifteenth years.

Socially integrated autistic children repeatedly present us with two characteristics. Firstly, a certain objectivity in their judgment of the world and other people, which is not very flexible but gives them a kind of unerring character. Secondly, an unusual measure of self-recognition and also self-limitation once they have reached their eighteenth or nineteenth year of life. This signifies a raised consciousness concerning their own actions, and limited insight in relation to the wide range of human needs and experiences. Such children do not enter certain situations if insight tells them that they could not cope.

In conclusion, based on the present extent of our experience, in practice as well as in theory, our point of departure is the assumption that all autistic children who come to us are searching for their own individual destiny in life. There is not much sense in hastily devising teaching models or therapeutic plans with the promise of general significance. The early diagnosis of autistic children is of particular importance and allows us to discuss the situation with parents before the obsessional circle of the autistic situation arises. More institutions ought to be established which would make it possible for autistic children to have opportunities out of their accustomed settings. Finally, we consider it urgently necessary that every autistic child receives

251

special schooling and therapy. Schools should be established along the lines of a curative educational school, where it is possible to offer children a wide variety of therapeutic and social activities.

I believe autistic children will find their place in society if we are prepared to accept that we are always dealing with special children with their own individual destiny, not only the autistic syndrome. Such an insight is an effective therapeutic precondition for all curative educational activity.

Part Two

Taken from a lecture to special needs educators at the Paedagogical Institute, Düsseldorf, under the title, Special Educational Aspects for the Development of Autistic Children. First published in the papers of the Paedagogical Institute, Düsseldorf, Volume 35, November 1977.

We are still actively engaged in finding new curative educational approaches for autistic children. We have been fortunate in being able to accompany a great number of autistic children for a fairly long period of time, and to follow their paths through school. Some areas will now be highlighted where it is important to recognise the specific disturbances of autistic children to help them by means of curative education.

We are unanimous here in understanding that the symptoms shown by autistic children are linked with perceptual disturbances and with the co-ordination and processing of different fields of perception. It is generally assumed that a person absorbs all kinds of sensory impressions, which are then built up into perceptions, by an essentially hidden mechanism localised in the brain. Here we find a subtle working together of activities of will, experiences of feeling and cognitive structuring. Inasmuch as they connect with every sensory perception, these activities need to facilitate a meaningful interpretation of the world. This is of great significance for the teacher, who must not overlook the fact that perceptions by the senses are active achievements. We cannot assume that we are passively conditioned through sensory experiences, but rather that we ourselves have to actively connect the sense perceptions as relational experiences with each other. This active relating of sensory perceptual fields through the ego and its organisation appears to be disturbed or limited in autistic children. The establishing of inter-relationships is dependent on perceptual judgments, so we should ask which sensory fields are in question here?

Firstly, there is the field of seeing (sight). Other sensory perceptions such as smelling, tasting and, indirectly, hearing also belong to this middle field. We also have a second sensory field, which plays an especially important role in the treatment and education of autistic children. It relates to our balance and our movement, whereby we contend with the earth's forces of gravity. We are dealing here with the ability to sense movement. With autistic children we find an obvious severe disturbance in this whole field of own body experience related to the four lower or body senses (touch, life, movement and balance). Following from this, we also find severe disturbances in autistic children's own identity with the body. This arrives early on for normal children, who build up body schemata from experiencing through the senses of movement and balance.

There is also a third field of perception, which is not acknowledged by present-day science as a primary sensory realm. This is particularly regrettable because it presents an obstacle for the understanding of autistic children. This is the field where a person's attention is directed to the soul-spiritual nature of another human being; to their speaking, thinking and behaviour or, more precisely, to the intentions evident in their behaviour. If you observe the disorders in speech perception in these children you will discover that their problems of communication, imitation and non-perception of the social environment are based on a difficulty in developing this higher sensory field.

If our understanding of speech is limited to a secondary or symbolic processing of perceptions, then we will be limited in what we can do to help autistic children. Indeed, we may well produce the opposite results from what we actually hope to achieve! If our concept of speech fails to include the speaker and their intentions, we will be equally limited.

We have autistic children who treat speech like an object; they listen and repeat what they hear but do not relate the spoken word to the speaker. This means that they are unable to understand what speech reveals about another person.

Normally young children are able to directly perceive the being, speech and thought of another person. If these inter-human fields of perception are not sufficiently available, as is the case with autistic children, they suffer a continuous collapse, or lack of development, in terms of their own experience of identity. Robbed of their own sense of identity, autistic children have to invent all kinds of things – maintenance of sameness in their spatial surroundings, etc. – in order to achieve at least one semblance of security in the world.

From a pedagogical point of view it is essential that we educate in the three fields of lower, middle and higher senses. Motor-sensory training alone might be of some help, but its application is still far from fully addressing the real problem of the interaction of the three sensory fields, in which the whole personality is involved, not only the functioning of the brain.

For example, an autistic child is piecing together a jigsaw puzzle, and you address that child. You may have the impression the child is deaf. You might experience a similar situation if you are intensely absorbed in something and somebody talks to you. In this instance what is seen in an extreme form in the autistic child is not dissimilar to our normal experience.

In order to perceive the world normally, through our senses, we have to be able to perform active transformation; we have to wrest ourselves away from our field of action and turn towards the perceptual space available for listening and speech, in order to perceive the other human being. Otherwise we cannot understand.

The ability to change from one sensory field to another is not yet developed at birth. In fact children gain this transformational ability to combine the three sensory fields around the third year of life. With autistic children we must exercise these transformative powers to make the co-ordination of the sensory fields possible. The result of this co-ordination is signified essentially by the child learning to say 'I' with regard to self. With an autistic child, we can say we have succeeded in this when he is able to relate the words 'I am' to himself.

Teachers have observed that, when asked to follow a line or lines drawn on paper or engraved in wood, with a pencil, finger or eye control, autistic children do less well than normal children. However, the moment autistic children are asked to perform the same task blindfold, they show extraordinary speed and skill, superior to that of normal children using sight. However, autistic children have a much reduced latitude of freedom to modify their movements and to experience themselves as a self in their activity. From this example we can see how co-ordination from the lower sensory field, the sense of movement, is not sufficient here to accompany information from the sense of sight, belonging to the middle field. This presents a lack of perceptual rhythm between two different fields, a rhythm which is available to normal children, giving them the basis for self-consciousness in their activities.

An autistic child can do a jigsaw puzzle with extraordinary speed, which is unobtainable for a normal child. The picture guide does not contribute to the process because autistic children cannot co-ordinate movement and seeing. Autistic children are riveted only to the spatial patterns of their activity. We are dealing here not with a deficit in a single sensory field, but with a co-ordination disorder. The picture of the jigsaw puzzle is quite irrelevant for autistic children; only the shapes are relevant and how they fit together. Inner mobility between two sensory fields (what above we have called transformation) is disturbed in a particular and specific way. This has considerable consequences for the special educational treatment of these children. If you fail to bring about the relationship of movement to sight, you do not actually help children, and exercises and skills then remain exterior to their personality development.

We know that a person gets dizzy if they turn round very quickly. When the movement stops they get a post-rotational nystagmus: the eyes continue moving, even though the body has stopped. This proves that, generally speaking, eye movement is linked with the movements of the entire organism. If one places an autistic child on a rotating chair and turns it fast, the autistic child will either not have a post-rotational nystagmus, or will experience a much shorter one than a normal child. It appears as if these children are only turned from the outside, and the own body, equilibrium experience plays no part; the body was merely an object that was turned round. We observe something similar with blind children.

Autistic children are subject to spatial determining factors with regard to their movement organism, without being able to co-ordinate their experiences with other sensory fields. There is even the danger that the other realms of the senses only relate symbiotically to the outer world of space. We can see this particularly in the fascination with mechanical-technical movements and programmed sequences in gadgets. Autistic children tend to merge in fascination with these movements and, again and again, start to perform these outer movements. These external movements have nothing to do with the child's own body experience of movement – through which experience of the motile world is constituted as perceptual judgment – but with external laws of physics. In consequence the child becomes passive and finally resigns from all self-initiative to move.

Related to this, we also see a decrease of motor achievements when a child is asked to do something. One can observe the dwindling or disintegration of stereotypical activities and notice that, to begin with, all is well. However, soon the movements turn into mechanical-stereotypical sequences of activity, which lack the transformation brought about through the optic field and through the perception of the other human being.

Something else, which is again connected with the co-ordination of the sensory fields, can be observed in the word-understanding of autistic children, connected with the higher senses. Autistic children run the risk of building up a certain space of activity around themselves, which another person cannot easily penetrate or enter into. The difficulty for autistic children is to establish a link between these two spaces of activity; to relate the space of activity of another person with their own space of activity.

This is one of the great difficulties at school: the fundamental problem of making contact. Autistic children do everything in a closed off space of activity and, when the teacher does something, it is alien to them; they are not able to build up a mutual space of activity with another human being. When, however, such disorders show themselves in very young children, we can therapeutically build a common, mutual space of activity. I believe there are various ways to do this, but it should not take the form of sitting opposite a child and demanding certain tasks. One has to allow children to accept something. For example, a child looks at an object, moves it and places it somewhere, then allows his therapeutic partner to take the same object and do something with it. Within such a rhythm of encounter, which you can also call play or a game, a meeting place between child and therapist is created.

All learning has to relate to a mutual common world, as the basis for relationships. If that is not the case, learning, imitation, acceptance and participation are not possible, and life consists of merely unrelated items. I see the establishment of a mutual world as an essential therapeutic task. Whether to establish this meeting space through purposely designed play, or by another means, should be left to the ingenuity of the therapist or teacher. However, it is quite obvious that one-to-one therapy sessions are necessary.

Although autistic children seemingly have no difficulty in perceiving objects, even being able to recognise and sometimes name them, they do not yet realise that this object is there simultaneously for another person, and that it is an object within the field of communication. This poses an important and central question in teaching and therapy, and much depends on how we think about it.

In order to awaken communicative activity in autistic children, teachers have to direct them towards inter-human sensory perceptions. If children do not understand someone else's intentions and you raise your voice to these children, they might retreat further still. This is not because they cannot understand what is spoken, but because the intentions inherent in speech or in the actions of other people are alien to them, or appear distorted or threatening. Every culture of any language is bound up with situations and spoken words which can only be understood when the intentions of the other person are perceived. I form within myself understanding of speech, in the moment I turn towards the words of the other person and I listen.

This has extraordinary consequences for lessons. It is not enough to speak to autistic children loudly and with good articulation; you also have to speak in simple language, leading children to listen actively in order to meet the intentions permeating your speech. You might have to whisper. What is at stake is your therapeutic attitude, which begins with teaching how to listen. To do this, teachers and therapists have to undergo training to develop the right attitude and correct insights regarding these higher sensory fields.

Normally in young children, a direct perception of the speech, thought and ego of another person takes place. Through our therapeutic attitude, we have to cultivate this activity of the higher senses in autistic children, in relation to the sense of movement, as one of the lower senses. It is important to help children, through certain exercises, to experience their own body. Every action of ours is a gesture, a symbolic presentation to which we give shape through our body. Gestures come about only when I can make free use of my body as an instrument; my ego finds expression through my body. The severe disorders of autistic children in this area are well-known: their inability to use the body as a means of expressing soul and spirit. Even if an autistic child learns to write, the child may not seem to be present in the activity. In such cases, therapeutic exercises can help. We try to dissolve the rigidity in their writing by letting them give shape to the same word or sentence in different forms: letting them write from right to left, or from above to below, or in a different style, or with different colours or materials, so that children slowly begin to experience joy in expression. What we call motivation for our actions does not only arise from being able to achieve something, such as writing a word or saying something, but also on how far we can inwardly experience something through our sense of life.

A child at play is not concerned with ruling the world or achievement, but with expression, which is experienced through movement. This experience, and the motivation related to it, is lacking in autistic children. We should, then, take care that children learn to experience joy, with which the ability to play is closely related. The sense of movement is linked to joy, as a body-soul quality. I have observed how autistic children, for the first time, jump freely in their surroundings, whereas before they darted to an object as if pulled by a string, or walked close to a wall with the most bizarre stereotypical movements. We give certain exercises, simple movements and balance exercises in eurythmy, with the aim that children should slowly inwardly perceive their own movements.

The phenomenon of joy and smiling is not dependent on complicated psychological mechanisms but rather, and especially with small children, simply on the unfolding of the sense of movement and the related ability to move freely and playfully. From this, we can see what a great store of sensory experiences, reaching into the soul, is transmitted to the human being from the realm of lower or body senses (König 1986).

During the course of autistic children's education, their symptoms not only change, but they also undergo development like any other child. The symptoms we find in autistic children prevent their personalities from sufficiently revealing themselves. Our task is to see a fixed pattern of activity and perception as a symptom, and to help children so that their personalities can unfold more freely.

Autistic children need many years of education, extending into adulthood, during which they can learn continuously. The suffering of autistic children is usually greatest during the first seven years of life. During the second seven years, many autistic children gain certain thinking abilities and learn gradually to cope with their discrepancies from the norm. They do not become normal, but they can learn to master their difficulties. You can, for example, observe autistic children of nine or ten years old who still have an obsession but, with curative education, learn to build up inter-human connections and gain some distance from their obsessions. A sense of humour may also develop. The child still has to run around the table before sitting down, but you have the impression that this is no longer a completely dominant ritual: the child could almost dispense with it. An intimate tendency of inner liberation from obsession becomes evident. Such observations are important because they show starting points for further educational and therapeutic progress.

During the third seven years of life, if autistic youngsters are cared for in a curative educational setting, important developmental steps can still occur, especially in the domain of human relationships. Much patience is required in supporting these children. One should not count on quick success. Above all, we have to consider the time factor in the development of a personality, and be aware of the maturing of the three sensory fields.

In conclusion, reference should be made to the intelligence of autistic children. Comprehensive research has shown that these children have a special kind of intelligence in certain fields, which is generally considered to be visual-spatial. We have already said that autistic children have an extraordinary, but pathological affinity to the physical-spatial world and its laws, which are extracted from the spatial conditions of the world during the first seven years of life through experiences of movement and balance (see Chapter 13). From this we can understand how autistic children are able, quite early on, to develop formal conceptual structures, leading to abstract yet impersonal thought activity. During the second seven-year period you can follow this process step by step. You also see the severe lack of an imaginative kind of thinking, which should come about through normal inter-human fellowship and the ability to imitate. Linked to these imaginative conceptions in a normal child is the ability to remember images; that is, a biographical long-term memory. This is disturbed in autistic children with deep consequences.

In autistic children we can see the premature intrusion and perception of the outer world of space, and a progression to conceptual, impersonal formulations, sometimes already during the first seven-year period. We notice that these children have the increasing tendency to translate everything into spatial terms, even in their verbal structures and expressions. They lack the time-related mobility of free creative thinking, and with it the ability to tune in to the thoughts of other human beings. Therefore we often have the impression that autistic children are very clever. This cleverness however pertains only to the area of formal structures, as developed by physical science. We find a kind of technical-formal intelligence which, in normal child development, should only arise after imaginative thinking has developed, so that during the second and third seven-year periods the two can harmonise with each other.

We therefore have to educate autistic children early, and in the right way, because the age at which inter-human connections are formed is during the period of imitation, namely, the first seven years. The age at which technical intelligence emerges in normal children is around the age of fourteen, when they tackle the laws of physics and mechanics.

In autistic children this development is reversed, because they are bound to an exterior world which can only be put into context in a formal and logical manner. At the same time, they suffer a severe lack of speech and thought formation from their deficit of inter-human development. This discrepancy becomes a central problem at school. The formal thought structures of autistic children are obsessional, schematic and rigid, and serve to provide a pseudo-security of an impersonal kind. In contrast to the free thought of older, normally developed children, the thoughts of autistic children are not free, but are a means to cope with the spatial world of perception. They are, therefore, bound up with many phobias.

People only develop secure personalities through a balance between imaginative and formal intelligence. With a number of autistic children, engaging them creatively in crafts and in more general work provides a great opportunity to foster and establish inter-human connections; especially when they have reached some degree of freedom in formal thinking. Nevertheless, their experience of the world remains still predominantly co-ordinated according to geometrical, mathematical and physical structures.

Lastly, our experiences in curative education show how important it is for autistic children to work in small classes, and to have regular individualised therapies. A rhythm can be established between individual therapy and group teaching which meets the special needs of each child.

15. Curative Educational Therapy: Exercises in the Realm of the Four Body Senses

First published in German under the title 'Neue Aspekte der Förderung Autistischen Kinder,' in *Autismus Heute Volume 2*, Verlag Modernes Lernen, Dortmund (1990).

The exercises described in the following account are based on the recognition that the lower senses of touch, movement, life and balance not only play an essential role in the development of communication with the external world in early childhood, but are also the basis of the functional development of other senses, such as hearing and seeing.

During the first seven years, children increasingly experience their own body, which defines its limits *vis-à-vis* the environment and surrounding forces, and thereby they establish a sense of ego-identity in space. During this stage the maturing lower body senses shape children's experience of their own body form or body image. This dimension of a developing own world, disturbed in autistic children, can be diagnosed in detail.

As autistic children do not actively relate to the world through touching, experiencing gravity or perceiving the formative forces in the world around them, they cannot sufficiently develop their own body experience as the basis of communication. The body, therefore, is not available as an adequate locus for the processing of other sensory experiences, such as hearing and seeing. Normal development of an inner gestalt, or body schemata, is underdeveloped and impeded in autistic children, and this is exemplified in their inability to imitate. Disorders in the field of the four lower senses in autistic children are evident in:

1. The relationship to organic substances (nutritional and digestive problems).
2. The relationship of own movement patterns to the environment: on the one hand stereotypical movements and, on the other hand, a dependency on external prompts.
3. The avoidance of experiences through touch and exploration.
4. The realm of gravity: the retreat into stereotypes and rituals, and compulsive dependency on spatial positioning.

With these patterns of behaviour, autistic children are manifesting an attempt – through ritualised and compulsive means – to uphold their identity. Such attempts constitute behaviour that we term autistic, and represent the phenomenology of failed communication.

The following exercises, initiated mainly by a partner, have proved effective in practical work with autistic children at the residential special school of Brachenreuthe (a Camphill residential school in Southern Germany).

The therapeutic task within the exercises is the stimulation of the child's own will-activity (intentionality), however basic it might appear, to provide a precondition for the gradual process of meaningful bodily experience, which will counter stereotypes, rituals and spatial compulsions.

Resistance exercises

These stimulate children coming to terms with the forces of gravity and experiencing themselves as independent and able to stand on their own feet. By means of such exercises the sense of balance in movement is exercised by overcoming gravity in the environment, which is done (under normal circumstances) when children learn to walk, and in grasping, moving or carrying objects.

Retarded interplay with the earth-gravity space is indicated by ritualistic movements, extremely lax muscle tone, walking on tiptoes, retarded explorative grasping (especially of heavy objects), as well as pathological movement patterns and stereotypes in walking and running. Therefore we introduce a sense of gravity to children by means of medicine ball games; exercises with hand weights; balancing; also using lead-weighted anklets to enhance resistance through gravity; carrying heavy objects; carrying out partner resistance exercises to make children aware of their own body weight. In the course of such planned daily exercises the following can soon be noticed: activating muscle tone; increasing surety of own body experience; decreasing spatial compulsions; better grip and eye contact.

Through strengthening children's body experience in this way they realise, 'I can keep myself within the space in which I stand and walk. I remain always the same wherever I am in space and, with this experience, I can judge the spatial situation of the world and of things.'

General movement exercises

We know that autistic children fail to imitate; that early on in the development of body movement, the transition from reflexes to imitation fails to take place sufficiently. This results in stereotypical movements with or without objects, and sometimes weak muscle tone. Own movement impulses cannot be implemented, nor can they be planned. The movements of these children are dependent on alien movements with which they like to identify, and also with being passively moved.

We endeavour therapeutically to build up self-experience in movement via the sense of movement. To begin with, meaningful movements in eurythmy are undertaken, which correspond to the sounds of speech. We do this together with children at first, possibly from behind, until they begin to relate and, eventually, start to imitate spontaneously. Children learn to sense extension and contraction, fast as opposed to slow movement, and resistance, and gradually learn through elementary eurythmy to acquire the full scale of human movement. Through such exercises, joy often appears, sometimes for the first time expressing a sense of own movement within the world, but also often for the first time, expressing the experience of: 'I can achieve something in the world.' In eurythmy therapy, special exercises are prescribed by a medical doctor, which work on the bodily formative processes, including the functioning of organs. Through such exercises autistic children can gain own body experiences. These experiences can also be achieved by exercising left and right, up and down, behind and in front, and different types of walking. The connection of eurythmy exercises with the sounds of speech stimulates the formation of the inner gestalt that underlies speech, and opens up new possibilities of response through imitation (Klimm 1981).

Many autistic children have problems with the development of dominance. This manifests not only in stereotypical symmetrical movement, but also in disturbed walking. Target exercises with bow and arrow, fencing in its traditional form, as well as exercises such as catching and throwing a rod with one hand, have proved useful. These exercises promote the asymmetry of the movement organisation against the symmetrical tendency in the structure and function of the head and central nervous system.

The sense of life

A disturbed sense of life in children requires special attention and manifests in a number of noticeable symptoms, such as the refusal to eat, disturbed meal rhythms or compulsive preferences for food with a particular appearance or consistency, as well as metabolic and body-building problems, which are often of a chronic nature. Besides medical treatment of digestive activity, special attention should be given to a regular daily rhythm of eating, as well as the soul shelter required in the eating environment. Children should learn, in due course, to accept all different kinds of food. Application of certain ointments, and baths with herbal supplements, can also help. Children are often helped by a slight shading of the dining room as well as by a dark red basic wall colouring. Small, even tiny portions are an essential starting point with eating difficulties, in order to stimulate the child's self-activity, which is important with all measures taken at the level of the body senses.

Touch exercises

We let the children look for an object in warmed sand or discriminate between several objects in sand by touching. We also exercise explorative touching without eye contact of two-dimensional shapes, which can be made of plywood, as a pre-exercise for visual exploration of letters and other forms. We use the same forms for children to walk or draw with their feet in sand, in order that one and the same phenomenon becomes reality for children in different sensory media. Encouraging children to touch parts of their own body and those of the therapist exercises, primarily, the demarcation of their own body as distinct from another.

Such touch exercises are important because the earliest boundary experience of one's own body *vis-à-vis* the material world is gained through touching. This normal development is delayed or disturbed in autistic children, and communicative and active exploration of the environment can only take place, and touch-oversensitivity retreat, when the sense of touch is activated. Then the personal body integrates into the existential substance of the world and children experience other bodies as objects in their own right.

The curative educator has every opportunity to discover new exercises within the parameters described here. Further exercises are described in *Sensory Integration and the Child* by A.J. Ayres, whose remarks regarding autistic children are helpful, and partly supplement what has been stated here.

Which particular exercises to do with an individual autistic child is always a new discovery and does not require a specialist therapist.

However, one must be able to work daily with the child, one-to-one in a quiet room.

Play and imitation

Play can be based on sensory exercises or it can supplement them, according to the developmental stage of the child. The aim is to further the child's imitation by dealing with objects in partnership. Firstly, we position ourselves at a table with playthings, behind or next to the child, and encourage him to respond using mobile objects, such as marbles. Soon the child joins in playing, using his own initiative. Then the therapist can move to sit opposite the child. Instead of mobile objects, others are now introduced, such as toy bricks, and in partnership some construction is undertaken, a tower or a bridge. Rhythm is very important, and the therapist should say, 'I place a brick, you place a brick, I place a brick,' until the tower is built. This mutual play is accompanied by speech and, in turn, challenges the own activity of the child. It is important that the child experiences that objects can stand together in space in different positions – next to, above, beneath, behind, in front – and that the child can be guided to establish these different and changing spatial positions with the same objects. The aim of these exercises is to see that the object remains the same in various spatial situations, never mind whether it is moved by the child or therapist. This realisation is preliminary to forming concepts. The mutual and alternating passing of objects, and the child's acceptance of this reciprocal action, are often necessary preliminary exercises to playing. The fundamental aim is to set imitation in motion and to establish a mutual world of objects.

Exercises in the listening space

These exercises aim to enhance a more wakeful ability to perceive tone. Diagnostically, autistic children's problems in the acoustic field are shown in delayed participation in group singing and, especially, in the detailed and rigid rendering of once-heard rhythms and melodies, which can take on a compulsive character and be used as a defense strategy in stressful situations.

This shows children's inability to synchronise perception and memory of what has been heard, because autistic children are not sufficiently able to respond to music directly through movement (muscle tone). Tone eurythmy has particularly shown its worth, as the heard musical elements (pitch, duration, rhythm) are performed by children through movement within the directions of space.

Children can thereby learn to experience themselves in tone eurythmical movement, actively reaching to overcome their dependencies and fixations. These exercises have proved particularly positive for children and adolescents during and after puberty, as has country dancing.

We conduct these exercises in the frame of tone eurythmy group lessons, but also as tone eurythmy therapy single lessons. By uniting the heard music with movement, frozen musical memories can be released, and the perceptive ability and openness of the child's movement organism for music is refreshed and developed. With another therapy exercise, also done individually, we have good results with autistic children with slack muscle tone and whose oversensitivity to tone and noise is a noticeable symptom. In tone eurythmy, children learn movement gestures for the intensity of tones, to counter the strong musical tones produced, for example, by a trumpet. It is important for autistic children that, within the sensory field of hearing and rhythm, balance is achieved between under- and oversensitivity. It becomes evident that this relationship is essentially dependent on the movement organisation and related muscle tone condition. In listening space therapy, we try to harmonise the interrelationship between listening and moving. This is an essential pre-exercise for furthering autistic children's interest in the sounds of speech.

Another exercise in this field is improvised musical conversations, where the therapist speaks to children with tone phrases on the lyre, and children are encouraged to answer freely on their instrument. Such tone conversations have the power to undo the pathological habit, in some autistic children, of talking to themselves, which prevents spontaneous communication owing to the preponderance of rigid memories.

When autistic symptoms begin to show in earliest childhood, the lyre (a string instrument) has proved effective. Young children accept instrumental music, which is tuned in with the rhythmic organisation, more easily than speech. One can also here accompany the sounding of tones with movement impulses. (Not passive moving but stimulating the child's own movement-intentions, through gentle muscular massage or touching.)

All these exercises are directed at further developing the connection between listening and movement organisation, as the basis of perceptual interest and processing of hearing perceptions. Stereotyped fixation of movement and slack muscle tone are outer signs of a disturbed relationship that can lead to a high degree of aversion or avoidance within the acoustic realm, including speech. Such avoidances in the auditory field have similar cause and effect as the avoidance of eye contact in the visual. These children are unable to engage exploratively in aspects of time or sequence, of what was seen or heard. Therefore they are often diagnosed as hearing impaired.

Warmth therapies

Among the therapies we have successfully applied are controlled temperature, or pyrogenic, baths. These stimulate the warmth organisation of autistic children and have proved successful in other institutions (Klimm 1981). Physically, autistic children are, by nature, cold. We apply oil dispersion baths or simple temperature-increase baths with an increase of one or two degrees centigrade above the child's body temperature. During and after such applications children make better eye contact and, in speaking children, their speech is activated and they can communicate better with simple games and imitation. Similar effects can also be seen with warm foot baths in the morning, followed by rubbing until the feet become pink. Such foot baths in the evening help children who have problems falling asleep.

Through regular therapy of this kind, continued for some months, the ego of the child can learn to establish itself within the peripheral warmth organisation, and thereby lay the foundation for soul expressions.

However, all measures described here can only become effective with autistic children and adolescents when seen within the framework of other social, curative educational and special educational approaches. A constitutional medical therapy also belongs here, using potentised medicines on the basis of an anthroposophically extended art of healing.

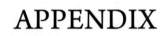

APPENDIX

1. Additional Anthroposophic Background

Rudolf Steiner and anthroposophy

Steiner described in detail how to embark on this 'path of knowledge', both in his fundamental books (Steiner 1973, 1989 & 1993) and in various lecture cycles (Steiner 1969a, 1978 & 1990a). It is clear from these that the conscientious study of anthroposophy constitutes the first, essential step on this path towards higher knowledge.

In 1925, from the viewpoint of the spiritual investigator, he wrote:

> The subject-matter of his exposition, namely the realities of the world of spirit, will be cast into forms of thought which the prevailing consciousness of our time – scientifically thoughtful and wide-awake, though unable to see into the spiritual world – can understand. (Steiner 1989, 8)

Environmental factors

In anthroposophy, the profound formative importance given to early imitation has not been lessened by current views that fail to see this capacity as a key feature of child development (Sylva & Lunt 1982). However, it has to be understood that with regard to imitation, Steiner did not simply mean the mere copying of the behaviour of others. He pointed to a very subtle process of active internalisation that works covertly into the finer organic constitution of the child: '...the human being during the first period of life inwardly reproduces all that is happening around him' (Steiner 1988, 50).

Steiner said that everything in the way of movement and gesture is inwardly reproduced by young children, and it is precisely because infants literally sleep and dream their way into earthly life that they are such natural imitators and mimics. In early consciousness they are effectively at one with all that is around them.

> When a child enters physical existence he only continues
> the experiences he had in the spiritual world prior to
> conception ... There we are imitators to a much higher
> degree because we are united with the (spiritual) beings
> we imitate ... Benefit for a child is all the greater the more
> he is able to live not in his own soul but in those within
> his environment. (Steiner 1969b, 13)

If Steiner is indeed correct we must therefore see in imitation that power which already leads us, as infants, instinctively into the realm of inter-human relationships and social reciprocity.

The first three years of life

From what has been written about child development (see Chapter 3) it is clear that anthroposophy sees the infant's experiential world as very different in quality from the adult's in the areas of consciousness, perception and conception. Unlike adults, during the first life period (from birth to the seventh year), the ego of the child is intensively involved in constructing its individualised physical body. According to Steiner, during the first two and a half years, this wisdom-filled ego activity is especially directed towards the refinement of the brain.

> The ego has to elaborate the brain into a more delicately
> complicated structure, in order that later on the human
> being will be able to think. During the first years of life the
> ego is very active. (Steiner 1976a, 87)

Moreover, anthroposophic research discovered that it is precisely through the activity of the ego that the three monumental milestones of child development – walking, talking and thinking – are achieved. These occur during the first three years while the child is functioning perceptually like a unified sense organ, and very differently from an adult. Indeed, children's very essence is of a perceptive and 'imitative susceptibility' (Kügelgen 1975), through which they are intimately aware of, and sensitive to, their human environment. Therefore, in contrast to later adult awareness, we can perceive the infant's consciousness as wide and peripheral, expansive and universal (Weihs 1984; König 1994). This enables a direct *living into* the souls of others, without the limitations imposed by the individual self-centredness of later childhood.

The sensory organisation

In order to appreciate the developmental role of perception more fully and exactly, we first have to look at anthroposophy's knowledge of the 'twelve senses' as described by Steiner (1981 & 1990b), and later by other anthroposophic authors (Soesman 1990; Aeppli 1993; Childs 1996). It is only through the functioning of our complicated multi-sensory organisation that as adults we can integrate ourselves experientially into daily life. If any one of our senses is impaired or lacking, we will suffer from some degree of sensory deprivation. According to Steiner (1990b), we have access to these distinct realms through our twelvefold sense organism; namely, there are three distinct orientations accessible via our complete sense organism:

- Our own corporeality
- Our natural environment
- Our specifically human, social surroundings

For each of these three realms or fields of perception, a group of four senses is normally available. The twelve senses divide into three groups, as follows:

1. Four *body* or *lower* senses of touch, life, movement and balance to perceive our own corporeality (our body).
2. Four *soul* or *middle* senses of smell, taste, sight and warmth, to perceive our natural environment.
3. Four *spiritual* or *higher* senses of hearing, word, thought and ego, to perceive our human, social surroundings.

This threefold ordering of the twelve senses can also be seen in relationship to the three soul forces of thinking (spiritual or higher senses), feeling (soul or middle senses), and willing (body or lower senses).

Whereas the higher senses function on the level of *awake* conscious cognition, the lower senses, in polar contrast, belong to the level of the *sleeping*, unconscious will processes. In between, the middle senses function on the level of *dreaming* feelings (Aeppli 1993). Therefore, we can also call the four higher senses the *cognitive* senses, and the four lower senses, the *will* senses.

It would need a specific research volume in order to comprehensively describe the physiology, functioning, genesis and development of these twelve senses. Yet, even without this, it is clear that Steiner's extension of the sense organism, beyond the customary five senses, is of great significance for any holistic understanding of the human being and for developmental psychology.

Early motor and sensory developments

We are now in a position to consider normal sensory and motor developments that occur during the first three years of life, so that we can recognise incisive steps of incarnation which result in the child becoming both self-conscious and socially interactive.

The four lower senses unfold and function during the first year of life (Aeppli 1993, 45). It is likely that the *sense of touch* operates even before birth, and is afterwards stimulated by the care-giving and hands-on bodily contact that takes place, especially with the mother, and also through continual contact with immediate physical surroundings.

The *sense of life* is developed through the repeated rhythms of feeding, sleeping, changing, and the vital processes of life, such as breathing, digestion, excretion, warming etc.

The *senses of movement and balance* develop as infants learn to co-ordinate, order and control their initially chaotic movement organism. Weihs (1984) called this 'the descent of motor control', beginning with the co-ordination of the eyes, head and neck, and extending via shoulders and arms into the trunk and lower limbs. In this way children quite literally *grow* down, head first, into their earthly body. Having passed through the stages of reaching out, sitting and crawling, this descent leads to children pulling themselves into an upright position, firstly with the aid of some object. They are at last able to stand unsupported and soon after launch into their first steps.

However, according to anthroposophy, babies and infants have not yet gained a centred self-consciousness, though their initially diffuse, peripheric awareness – consisting of merging sense perceptions and feelings – is increasingly *lit up* as the world becomes differentiated from their bodily self-experience: 'The upright posture alone causes the abyss to open between self and world, and this leads to the further acquisition of speech and thought' (König 1984, 19).

Babbling, as a precursor to proper speech, begins some time after the sixth month, reaching its peak by nine to ten months. It has been found to be universal in infants the world over (see Sylva & Lunt 1982).

At the end of the first year, together with uprightness and walking, the *sense of word* begins to function, and language can be perceived. According to König (1984), the development of this higher sense is a necessary prerequisite for speaking. As long as children babble they have not yet developed *word sense*. At around eighteen months, an important new developmental step is made.

> Suddenly and quite spontaneously, the child grasps the connection of things through names ... An immediate understanding for the word itself and its meaning is present ... This new understanding of the meaning of

words is due to the emergence of the sense of thought.
Concepts are now perceived and grasped. Thus a small
child does not think the meaning of words he acquires,
but perceives it through his senses. (König 1984, 38–98)

A striking example of the first functioning of the *sense of thought*
is shown in the remarkable case of Helen Keller, who was both blind
and deaf. When, at the age of seven, this sense awakened in her, she
perceived with joy and excitement that, 'Everything had a name,
and each name gave birth to a new thought' (Meadows 1986, 121).
Although children in their second year are typically walking, talking
human beings, they do not yet think consciously.

Self-consciousness

The normal acquisition of self-consciousness enables all experiences
in children's lives – perceptions, thoughts, feelings and deeds – to be
referred to this newly gained *self-hood,* to their own soul centre.

But now, the moment we use the word 'I', we have
become inhabitants of the earth. This moment is a
critical point in human development, and so is one of
the most difficult events in a child's life, a crossroads at
which many children falter and perish. Many autistic
and psychopathic children break down at this particular
point. (König 1994, 104)

Why should it be a 'most difficult' event? Precisely because, until
this moment in time, children are living in a dream-like consciousness
in which they are still closely connected to their spiritual, pre-birth
existence, where they had dwelt with (and in) more highly evolved
spiritual beings. This is best expressed by Steiner:

Whereas what we call the child's aura hovers around
it during its earliest years like a wonderful human and

superhuman power and, being really the higher part of
the child, is continued on into the spiritual world, at the
moment to which memory goes back, this aura sinks more
into the inner being of the child ... Henceforward the
consciousness is at every point brought into connection
with the external world. This is not the case with a very
young child, to whom things appear only as a surrounding
world of dreams. (Steiner 1970a, 6–7)

This 'world of dreams' is not in any way qualitatively inferior for
young children than their newly acquired earthly self-consciousness,
but rather it reflects the soul's closeness to its spiritual origins. As we
have already seen, the state of dreaming consciousness belongs to
the feeling realm of the soul, and lies between *awake thinking* and the
sleeping unconscious processes of the will. In this sense, the experience
of acquiring self-consciousness is, quite literally, an *awakening* from a
previous dream state.

Thinking and the sense of ego

In recent decades, much has been written about young children's
thought processes (Donaldson 1978; Wood 1988; Meadows 1983 &
1993). It is now considered that pre-school children are much more
cognitively able than was previously believed (Piaget 1982).

An anthroposophic understanding sees that the awakening to self-
consciousness in children during the third year, and the awakening
to thinking as a real cognitive activity, go hand in hand (König 1984;
Lievegoed 1987). This is quite distinct from the functioning of the
sense of thought at around eighteen months. Both stem from the
encounter of dreaming children with something of their own true
being. Then, with the new age of defiance that emerges strongly in
children after the birth of individual self-consciousness and thinking,
the *sense of ego* can also begin to function.

This special sense of the ego as the inner essence of another person
grows in its perceptive capacity until, at around the ninth or tenth

year, it reaches a certain maturity. At this age, too, children will once again meet something of their own spiritual being and, in consequence and contrast, achieve a strengthened earthly self-consciousness. This existential experience is often accompanied by feelings of undefined loneliness and separation from the child's spiritual origins, as the incarnation process continues further and deeper into the physical bodily organisation (Koepke 1989).

The social context

Early child development takes place through interaction with others:

> Children are born into a complex social world: from
> infancy on, they are active participants in a world of other
> people – adults and children, familiar and not-so-familiar
> others. (Dunn 1988, 2)

Moreover, it has been observed that, 'During the first few months of life, the baby is fascinated by the world of people' (Karmiloff-Smith 1994, 202).

There are, therefore, clear early indicators that a child is destined to become a social being; to become both a recipient of, and a contributor to, the human community. However, children come to this social context already bearing certain seeds and intentions for the future, which, given favourable conditions, germinate and unfold over the course of time. Foremost amongst these necessary conditions will be the development of reciprocal relationships and interactions.

> These gifts and potentials can only be awakened when
> the surrounding world turns towards the child ... because
> a child will become nothing without the world of human
> beings. (König 1994, 91)

The neonate, infant and young child must be able to establish active contact and communication with their social human surroundings so that developmental processes, involving metamorphosis and transformation on different levels, can underpin their successful incarnation.

Two key concepts

Through new earthly incarnations, separated by intervening periods of intense activity spent in supersensible worlds of soul and spirit, the human being receives many opportunities by which to evolve to higher levels of development (Steiner 1973). This anthroposophic perspective is clearly the complete antithesis of any materialistic, evolutionary viewpoint that regards death as the end of individual consciousness and existence. However, it is also very different from any religious viewpoint that regards an afterlife (whether in heaven or hell) as the final destination and resting place of individual souls.

In particular, it is only through incarnation and ego-integration that each person can become a more moral and unselfish being, who carries co-responsibility for the progress of the world. This moral path of evolution can, however, only be exercised and gradually realised in the company of other people – in the active social milieu, not in individual solitude and isolation.

2. Further Therapies and Medical Treatments

Listening space therapy

The aim is to harmonise the interrelationship between listening and moving. Several children can be taken together in a room where visual stimuli are reduced; for example, there is dimmed lighting. The children move when music is played on a lyre, flute, and/or recorder. At first the music is composed of short, swift notes, and the children are encouraged to make quick forward steps in time to the music. Then some long notes are also played and the children move backwards slowly. Gradually, during the course of the session, the long, slow notes and the backward walking predominate, and this brings children to greater peace and an increased listening capacity. In the second part of the therapy, children sit and listen while music is played behind them. This therapy is particularly helpful for restless and hyperactive children, and pupils with autism can also benefit.

Trumpet therapy

In this therapy a number of children are guided to perform walking and eurythmy arm movements while tones are sounded. A trumpet is used to produce tones of increasing intensity. Children with autism can benefit because the therapy calls upon their own ego-forces to counter the strong trumpet sounds. This can also help to overcome any hypo-or hyper-sensitivity in hearing, due to a lack of ego-integration.

Riding therapy

According to Hansmann (1992), horse-riding therapy, as developed in curative education, is helpful for a broad spectrum of pupils including those who are autistically withdrawn. A certain relationship with music therapy exists, since the horse walks at a 4/4 rhythm, trots in a 2/2 rhythm and canters in a 3/4 rhythm. Riding helps to regulate a child's breathing rhythm and thus supports the flow of speech.

The special relationship a child with autism can form with the horse is therapeutic in itself, and fosters inner security and confidence. If children with autism can actually learn to direct the horse in a good walking rhythm, this will bear witness to their increased ego-control and integration. Other significant benefits have also been clearly described (see Hansmann 1992).

Coloured light therapy

This therapy unites eurythmy, colour and music, and aims to harmonise the breathing process in children. Overall, it has a quietening and calming effect.

A group of children sit on one side of a large, semi-transparent screen, and watch the play of beautiful coloured shadows created from the movements performed by a eurythmist on the opposite side of the screen. The coloured light comes from daylight passing through coloured windows or celluloids, and the actual combination of colours can be controlled and varied during the therapy. This is accompanied by music, usually from a lyre.

Chirophonetics

In this therapy the therapist phonates a sound while simultaneously stroking a corresponding shape on to the child's back. This massage stroke represents the form of a breath in the mouth during articulation.

Originally, this therapy was meant for children who failed to develop speech at the appropriate age. However, chirophonetics is now not used exclusively in stimulating the speech impulse, but more generally:

> ...particularly in the treatment of autism, with its many unsolved questions. An autistic child does not have recourse to the possibilities which his speech organs offer, he or she avoids confrontation with others through speech, most particularly when one wants to entice such a child to speak ... However, as chirophonetics makes no active demands on the child, it was helpful in a number of cases, in stimulating the will to speak. (Baur 1993, xv)

This therapy can also stimulate the power of imitation, which is impaired in young children with autism (Baur 1992).

Useful Organisations

The National Autistic Society (NAS)
393 City Road
London EC1V 1NG
Tel 020–7833 2299
www.autism.org.uk
    In Wales: www.autism.org.uk/wales
    In Scotland: www.autism.org.uk/scotland

Autism Independent UK
(previously known as Society for the Autistically Handicapped or SFTAH)
Tel 01526–523 274
www.autismuk.com

Camphill Communities in England and Wales
www.camphill.org.uk

ESPA (Education and Services for People with Autism) Research
(previously known as The Autism Research Unit at the University of Sunderland)
www.espa-research.org.uk

European Co-operation in Anthroposophical Curative Education and Social Therapy
www.ecce.eu

Scottish Autism
(previously known as the Scottish Society for Autism)
www.scottishautism.org

Parents for the Early Intervention of Autism in Children (PEACH)
www.peach.org.uk

Autism Research Institute
www.autism.com

Gluten Free Casein Free (GFCF)
American website produced by parents and professionals
(some British products listed)
www.gfcfdiet.com

Other websites

Research Autism www.researchautism.net
National Institute of Mental Health www nimh.nih.gov
Autism Research Centre www.autismresearchcentre.com
Intensive Interaction www.intensiveinteraction.co.uk
Sensory Integration www.sensoryintegration.org.uk
NICE (National Institute for Health and Care Excellence)
www.nice.org.uk

Local organisations

Please note that there are other regional organisations in your local area who will also be able to help you. Contact your local library or Social Services for further details, or search online for 'Autism' and the name of your region or country.

Bibliography

Aarons, M. & Gittens, T. 1992. *The Handbook of Autism: A Guide for Parents and Professionals*. London and New York: Routledge.

Aeppli, W. 1986. *Rudolf Steiner Education and the Developing Child*. New York: Anthroposophic Press.

—. 1993 (2013). *The Care and Development of the Human Senses*. Edinburgh: Floris Books

Alvin, J. & Warwick, A. 1992. *Music Therapy for the Autistic Child*. Oxford University Press.

American Psychiatric Association. 2013. *Diagnostic and Statistical Manual of Mental Disorders*, Fifth Edition (DSM-5). American Psychiatric Publishing.

Arnim, G. von. 1986. Körperschema und Leibessinne. *In* König 1986.

Astington, J. W. 1994. *The Child's Discovery of the Mind*. London: Fontana.

Attwood, T. 1998. *Asperger Syndrome, a Guide for Parents and Professionals*. London: Jessica Kingsley.

Autism Research Review. 1995. 9 (4). San Diego: Autism Research Institute.

Autism Research Unit. 1991. *Therapeutic Approaches to Autism: Research and Practice*. London: National Autistic Society.

Autism Resource Center of Central Massachusetts. 2012. 'Proposed DSM-5 criteria for autism spectrum disorders'.

Autism Speaks. 2013a. 'Genetics and Genomics', from www.autismspeaks.org

—. 2013b. 'How is autism treated?', from www.autismspeaks.org

Axline, V. M. 1985. *Dibs in Search of Self*. Harmondsworth: Penguin Books.

Ayres, A. J. 1995. *Sensory Integration and the Child*. Los Angeles: Western Psychological Services.

Baird, G., Simonoff, E., Pickles, A., Chandler, S., Loucas, T., Meldrum, D. & Charman T. 2006. 'Prevalence of disorders of the autism spectrum in a population cohort of children in South Thames: the Special Needs and Autism Project (SNAP)'. *The Lancet*. 368 (9531). pp. 210–215.

Bang, J. M. (Ed). *A Portrait of Camphill: From Foundling Seed to Worldwide Movement*. Edinburgh: Floris Books

Baron-Cohen, S. & Bolton, P. 1993. *Autism, the Facts*. New York: Oxford University Press.

Baron-Cohen, S., Tager-Flusberg, H. & Cohen, D. (Eds). 1993. *Understanding Other Minds*. Oxford: Oxford University Press.

Baron-Cohen, S. & Wheelwright, S. 2004. 'The empathy quotient: an investigation of adults with Asperger syndrome or high functioning autism, and normal sex differences'. *Journal of Autism and Developmental Disorders*. 34 (2). pp. 163–175.

Barron, J. & S. 1993. There's a Boy in Here. London: Chapmans.

Baur, A. 1992. 'Chirophonetics'. *Curative Education and Social Therapy*. (1). pp. 10–12.

—. 1993. *Healing Sounds: Fundamentals of Chirophonetics*. Sacramento: Rudolf Steiner College Press.

Beck, V. & Beck, G. 1998. *Unlocking the Potential of Secretin*. San Diego: published on www.osiris.sunderland.ac.uk/autism/sec.htm

Bettelheim, B. 1967. *The Empty Fortress*. New York: Free Press.

Biesantz, H. & Klingborg, A. 1979. *The Goetheanum, Rudolf Steiner's architectural impulse*. London: Rudolf Steiner Press.

Blakeslee, S. November 19, 2002. 'A Boy, a Mother and a Rare Map Of Autism's World', from *The New York Times*, Los Angeles.

Bogdashina, O. 2003. *Sensory Perceptual Issues in Autism and Asperger Syndrome*. London and Philadelphia: Jessica Kingsley.

—. 2006. *Theory of Mind and the Triad of Perspectives on Autism and Asperger Syndrome*. London: Jessica Kingsley Publishers.

Bosch, G. 1962. *Der frühkindliche Autismus*. Berlin: Springer.

Bott, V. 1982. *Anthroposophic Medicine*. London: Rudolf Steiner Press.

Boucher, J. 2009. *The Autistic Spectrum*. London: Sage.

Boucher, J. & Scarth, L. 1977. 'Research and the teaching of autistic children', in Furneaux, B. and Roberts, B. *Autistic Children*. London: Routledge & Kegan Paul.

Bragge, A. & Fenner, P. 2009. 'The Emergence of the "Interactive Square" as an Approach to Art with Children on the Autistic Spectrum'. *International Journal of Art Therapy*. 14 (1). pp. 17–28.

Britz-Crecelius, H. 1979. *Children at Play, Preparation for Life*. Edinburgh: Floris Books.

Bundy A., Lane S. & Murray E. 2002. *Sensory Integration Theory and Practice*. Philadelphia: F.A Davis Company.

Caldwell, P. 2005. *Finding You Finding Me: Using Intensive Interaction to Get in Touch with People whose Severe Learning Disabilities are combined with Autistic Spectrum Disorder*. London: Jessica Kingsley Publishers.

—. 2007. *From Isolation to Intimacy*. London: Jessica Kingsley Publishers.

—. 2010. *Autism and Intensive Interaction*. London: Jessica Kingsley Publishers.

Caldwell, P. & Horwood, J. 2008. *Using Intensive Interaction and Sensory Integration*. London, Philadelphia: Jessica Kingsley Publishers.

Cameron, C. & Moss, P. 2011. 'Social Pedagogy: Current Understandings and Opportunities', in *Social Pedagogy and Working with Children and Young People*. London: Jessica Kingsley Publishers.

Cambell-McBride, N. 2004. *Gut and Psychology Syndrome*. Medinform Publishing.

Chepelina, E., Winkleman, Ch., D'Agostino, V., Menzinger, B., Gordon, J. & Henderson, T. 2009. *Guiding Vision Statement*. Aberdeen: Camphill Schools Aberdeen.

Childs, G. 1991. *Steiner Education in Theory and Practice*. Edinburgh: Floris Books.

—. 1996. *Five + Seven = 12 senses. Rudolf Steiner's Contribution to the Psychology of Perception*. Stroud: Fir Tree Press.

Christie, N. 1989. *Beyond Loneliness and Institutions*. Oxford: Norwegian University Press.

Clarke, R. P. June, 2010. 'Copy number variations are at best only marginal to autism causation', from www.autismcauses.info

Connor, M. & Ferguson-Smith, M. 1977. *Medical Genetics*. Oxford: Blackwell Science.

Connor, S. June 10, 2010. 'Autism and genetics: A breakthrough that sheds light on a medical mystery', from www.independent.co.uk

Courchesne, E. 1991. 'Neuroanatomic imaging in autism'. Pediatrics. (87). Part 2. *Supplement*. pp. 781–90.

Damasio, A. 1999. *The feeling of what happens: Body, Emotion and the Making of Consciousness*. London: Heinemann.

Davy, J. (Ed). 1975. *Work Arising from the Life of Rudolf Steiner*. London: Rudolf Steiner Press.

Delacato, C.H. 1974. *The Ultimate Stranger, the Autistic Child.* California: Academic Therapy Publications.

Dohan. 'Cereals and schizophrenia: data and hypothesis'. *Acta Psychiatr.* Scand. 42:125.

Doidge, N. 2007 *The Brain that Changes Itself.* London: Penguin Books.

Donaldson, M. 1978. *Children's Minds.* London: Fontana.

—. 1992. New edition. Harmondsworth: Penguin Books.

—. 1992. *Human Minds,* Penguin Books.

Dunn, J. 1988. *The Beginnings of Social Understanding.* Oxford: Basil Blackwell.

Ekstein, R. 1973. *Grenzfallkinder.* Munich & Basel.

Elgar, S. & Wing, L. 1981. *Teaching Autistic Children, Guidelines for Teachers No.5.* London: National Autistic Society.

Elliot, A. 1990. 'Adolescence and early adulthood: the needs of the young adult with severe difficulties'. In Ellis, K. (Ed). 1990. *Autism.*

Ellis, K. (Ed). 1990. *Autism, Professional Perspectives and Practice.* London: Chapman & Hall.

Emery, M. & Forest, L. 2004. 'Art Therapy as an Intervention for Autism'. *Art Therapy: Journal of the American Art Therapy Association.* 21 (3). pp. 143–147.

Engel, P. 1968. 'Movement patterns and behaviour'. Unpublished lecture. Camphill British Regional Conference, Thornbury. Sheiling School Library.

Erikson, E. H. July, 1968. 'Die Ontogenese der Ritualisierung'. Psyche 7.

Evans, M. and Rodger, I. 2000. *Healing for Body, Soul, and Spirit: an Introduction to Anthroposophic Medicine.* Edinburgh: Floris Books.

Farrants, W. 1988. *Camphill Villages.* UK: Camphill Press.

Feuser, G. 1980. *Autistische Kinder.* Solms-Oberbiel: Jarick.

Firth, G., Elford, H., Leeming, C. & Crabbe, M. 2008. 'Intensive Interaction as a Novel Approach in Social Care: Care Staff's Views on the Practice Change Process'. *Journal of Applied Research in Intellectual Disabilities.* 21. pp. 58–69.

Fischer, E. 1965. *Jahrbuch für Jugendpsychiatrie und ihre Grenzgebiete.* 4. Bern.

Flavell, J. H. 1985. *Cognitive Development.* Prentice-Hall.

Frankland, M. 1995. *Freddie the Weaver.* London: Sinclair-Stevenson.

Frith, U. 1989. *Autism, Explaining the Enigma.* Oxford: Basil Blackwell.

—. (Ed). 1991. *Autism and Asperger Syndrome*. New
York: Cambridge University Press.

Furneaux, B. & Roberts, B. 1979. *Autistic Children, Teaching, Community
and Research Approaches*. London: Routledge & Kegan Paul.

Garvey, C. 1991. *Play*. London: Fontana.

Glöckler, M. & Goebel, W. 1990 (2013 4th Edition). *A
Guide to Child Health*. Edinburgh: Floris Books.

Grandin, T. 2006. *Thinking in Pictures*. London: Bloomsbury Publishing.

—. June 2000. 'My Experiences with Visual Thinking
Sensory Problems and Communication Difficulties'.
Centre for Study of Autism. www.autism.org

Grandin, T. & Scariano, M. 1986. *Emergence Labelled
Autistic*. Belford: Ann Arbor Publishers Ltd.

Guardian readers & Ruth Spencer. March 1, 2013. 'Parents of children with
autism on what "a cure" means to them', from www.guardian.co.uk

Hansmann, H. 1992. *Education for Special Needs, Principles and
Practice in Camphill Schools*. Edinburgh: Floris Books.

Happé, F. 1994. *Autism, an Introduction to Psychological
Theory*. London: UCL Press Ltd.

—. Happe, F. June 2011. *Journal of the American Academy of Child
& Adolescent Psychiatry* (JAACAP). 50 (6). pp. 540–542.

Harris, J. C. 1995. *Developmental Neuropsychiatry*.
Volume II. Oxford University Press.

Harris, P. L. 1991. *Children and Emotion*. Oxford: Basil Blackwell.

Harwood, A. C. 1975. 'Threefold man'. In Davy, J. (Ed).
Work arising from the life of Rudolf Steiner.

—. 1982. *The Recovery of Man in Childhood*. New
York: Anthroposophic Press.

Hauschka, M. 1979. *Rhythmical Massage*. London: Rudolf Steiner Press.

—. 1985. *Fundamentals of Artistic Therapy: the Nature and Task
of Painting Therapy*. London: Rudolf Steiner Press.

Heider, M. von. 1995. *Looking Forward*. Stroud: Hawthorn Press.

Hobson, R. P. 1993. *Autism and the Development of
Mind*. Lawrence Erlbaum Associates.

Hocking, B. 1990. *Little Boy Lost*. London: Bloomsbury.

Holtzapfel, W. 1993. 'I drown in loneliness'. *Curative Education
and Social Therapy*. Issue I. Easter 1993. pp. 4–9.

—. 1995. *Children with a Difference*. East Grinstead: Lanthorn Press.

Horvath, K., Papadimitrou, J.C., Rabsztyn, A., Drachenberg, C. & Tildon, J. T. November 1999. 'Gastro-intestinal Abnormalities in Children with Autistic Disorder'. *Journal of Pediatrics*. 135 (5). pp. 559–563.

Howlin, P. 1994. 'Facilitated communication and autism; are the claims for success justified?' *Communication*. 28 (2). pp. 10–12.

ICD-10. 1993. *International Classification of Diseases*. Geneva: World Health Organisation.

Humphrey, N. & Parkinson, G. 2006. 'Research on Interventions for Children and Young People on the Autistic Spectrum: A Critical Perspective'. *Journal of Research in Special Educational Needs*. 6 (2). pp. 76–86.

Insel, T. March 29, 2012. 'Autism Prevalence: More Affected or More Detected?', from www. nimh.nih.gov

—. February 26, 2013. 'The Four Kingdoms of Autism', from www.nimh.nih.gov

International Molecular Genetics Study of Autism Consortium. Newsletter Number 2. April, 2000. www.well.ox.ac.uk/-maestrin/news2000.html

Isserow, J. 2008. 'Looking Together: Joint Attention in Art Therapy' *International Journal of Art Therapy*. 13 (1). pp. 34–42.

Jackson, R. (Ed). 2006. *Holistic Special Education: Camphill Principles and Practice*. Edinburgh: Floris Books

Jepson, B. & Johnson, J. 2007. *Changing the Course of Autism*. US: Sentient Publications.

Jones, G. & Jordan, R. 2008. 'Research Base for Intervention in Autism Spectrum Disorders'. In McGregor et al (Eds). *Autism*. Oxford: Blackwell Publishing.

Jordan, R. 1999. *Autistic Spectrum Disorders*. David Fulton Publishers.

—. 2005. 'Autistic Spectrum Disorders'. In Lewis, A. & Norwich, B. (Eds). *Special Teaching for Special Children?* UK: Open University Press.

Jordan, R. & Powell, S. 1990. *The Special Curricular of Autistic Children: Learning and Thinking Skills*. London: The Association of Head Teachers of Autistic Children and Adults.

—. 1995. *Understand and Teach Children with Autism*. John Wiley & Sons.

Kanner, L. 1943. 'Autistic disturbances of affective contact'. *Nervous Child 2*. pp. 217–50.

Karmiloff-Smith, A. 1994. *Baby it's You*. London: Ebury Press.

Kaufman, B. N. 1976. *Son-rise*. New York: Warner Books.

Kehrer, H. E. 1978. *Kindlicher Autismus*. Basel, Munich: S. Karger.

Kirchner, H. 1977. *Dynamic Drawing: its Therapeutic Aspect*. New York: The Rudolf Steiner School.

Kirchner-Bockholt, M. 1992. *Fundamental Principles of Curative Eurythmy*. London: Temple Lodge

Kirchner-Bockholt, M. 2004. *Foundations of Curative Eurythmy* Edinburgh: Floris Books

Klimm, H. June, 1965. 'Über die heilpädagogische Behandlung von Kindern mit autistischen Erscheinungen'. *Pro Infirmis*.

—. 1981. *Beobachtungen and Erwägungen beim Autimus, Der frühkindliche Autismus als Entwicklungsstörung*. Stuttgart: Freies Geistesleben.

Knivsberg, A. M., Reichelt, K. L. & Nodland, M. April, 1999. 'Autism spectrum disorders in children in mainstream classes'. A collection of papers from the conference held in the University of Durham.

Koepke, H. 1989. *Encountering the Self, Transformation and Destiny in the Ninth Year*. New York: Anthroposophic Press.

Konferenz for Curative Education & Social Therapy, Secretariat of (Ed). 1995. List of the Anthroposophic Homes, Schools, Workshops, and Village Communities for Curative Education and Social Therapy. Dornach.

König, K. 1960. *The Autistic Child I & II*. English Translation in Sheiling School Library. (In German in: Muller-Wiedemann et al. 1988.)

—. 1971. *Sinnesentwicklung und Leiberfahrung, Heilpädagogik aus anthroposophischer Menschenkunde – 5*. Stuttgart: Freies Geistesleben. (English Translation in Sheiling School Library.)

—. 1984 (2004). *The First Three Years of the Child*. Edinburgh: Floris Books.

—. 1986. *Sinnesentwicklung und Leiberfahrung*. Stuttgart: Verlag Freies Geistesleben.

—. 1989. *Being Human: Diagnosis in Curative Education*. UK: Camphill Press.

—. 1990. *Man as a Social Being, and the Mission of Conscience*. UK: Camphill Press.

—. 1994. *Eternal Childhood*. TWT Publications Ltd., on behalf of the Camphill Movement.

—2008. *Ita Wegman and Karl König: Letters and Documents.* Edinburgh: Floris Books
—2008 *Karl König: My Task.* Edinburgh: Floris Books
—2009. *The Child With Special Needs: Letters and Essays on Curative Education.* Edinburgh: Floris Books
König, K. et al. 1953. 'The treatment with Thalamus'. Camphill in-house publication.
König, K., von Arnim, G. & Herberg. 1978. *Sprachverständnis und Sprachenbehandlung.* Stuttgart: Verlag Freies Geistesleben.
Kügelgen, H. von. (Ed). 1975. *Understanding Young Children, Extracts from Lectures by Rudolf Steiner compiled for the use of Kindergarten Teachers.* London: Rudolf Steiner Press.
Lainhart, J. E. & Lange, N. November 9, 2011. 'Increased neuron number and head size in autism'. *The Journal of the American Medical Association,* from www.jamanetwork.com
Lauer, H. E. 1977. *Die zwölf Sinne des Menschen.* Schaffhausen.
Leaning, B. & Watson, W. 2006. 'From the Inside Looking Out: An Intensive Interaction Group for People with Profound and Multiple Learning Disabilities.' *British Journal of Learning Disabilities.* 34 (2). pp.103–9.
Le Breton, M. 1996. *Diet Intervention and Autism.* London: Jessica Kindersley.
Ledford, H. June 9, 2010. 'Rare genetic variants linked to autism', from www.nature.com
Lewis, L. 1998. *Understanding and Implementing Special Diets to Aid in the Treatment of Autism and Related Developmental Disorders.* Future Horizons Inc.
Lievegoed, B. 1987 (2005). *Phases of Childhood.* Edinburgh: Floris Books.
—. 1993. *Phases, the Spiritual Rhythms of Adult Life.* Bristol: Rudolf Steiner Press.
Lovell, A. 1978. *Simple Simon: the Story of an Autistic Boy.* Lion Publishing.
Lutz, C. 1968. *In Müller-Wiedemann et al 1988.* Der frühkindliche Austismus.
Luxford, M. 1994 (2006). *Children with Special Needs; Rudolf Steiner's Ideas in Practice.* Edinburgh: Floris Books.
Mahler, Margaret S. 1968. *On Human Symbiosis and the Vicissitudes of Individuation: Infantile Psychosis.* Connecticut. International Universities Press.

—. 1995. 'Infantile Psychosis'. *Selected Papers of Margaret S. Mahler. Volume 1.* New Jersey: Jason Aronson.

Martin, N. 2009. 'Art Therapy and Autism: Overview and Recommendations'. *Art Therapy Journal of the American Art Therapy Association.* 26 (4). pp. 187–190.

McAllen, A. 1999. *The Extra Lesson.* Fair Oaks CA: Rudolf Steiner Press.

Meadows, S. 1983. *Developing Thinking: Approaches to Children's Cognitive Development.* London & New York: Methuen.

—. 1986. *Understanding Child Development.* London: Unwin Hyman.

—. 1993. *The Child as Thinker.* London & New York: Routledge.

Melzer, P. July 11, 2008. 'Autism and Genes Revisited', from Pete's Blog, brainmindinst.blogspot.com/2008/07/autism-genes-revisited.html

Miedzanik, D. 1986. *My Autobiography.* University of Nottingham, Child Development Research Unit.

Müller-Wiedemann, H. 1966. 'Social development in handicapped children'. In Pietzner, C. *Aspects of Curative Education.* Aberdeen: Aberdeen University Press.

—. June 14–21,1982. *Autism and Ego-Development.* Unpublished notes from three lectures given in Camphill, Scotland. Sheiling School Library.

—. 1990. Neue Aspekte der Förderung autistischer Kinder. In *Autismus Heute.* Vol. 2. Dortmund: Verlag Modernes Lernen.

Müller-Wiedemann, H., König, K., Weihs, T. J. *et al.* 1988. *Der frühkindliche Autismus als Entwicklungsstörung.* Stuttgart: Freies Geistesleben.

Murray-Slutsky, C. & Paris, B. 2000. *Exploring the Spectrum of Autism and Pervasive Developmental Disorders.* The Psychological Corporation USA.

NICE Guideline on Recognition, Referral, Diagnosis and Management of Adults on the Autism Spectrum (National Clinical Guideline). 2012. National Collaboration Centre for Mental Health. London: RCPsych Publications.

Niederhäuser, H.R. & Frohlich, M. 1974. *Form Drawing.* New York: Rudolf Steiner School.

Nind, M. 1996. 'Efficacy of Intensive Interaction.' *European Journal of Special Needs Education.* 11. pp. 48–66.

Nind, M. & Hewett, D. 1994. *Access to Communication: Developing the basics of communication with people with severe learning difficulties through Intensive Interaction.* London: David Fulton

—. 2001. *A Practical Guide to Intensive Interaction.* Kidderminster: British Institute of Learning Disabilities.

—. 2008. *Access to Communication*. UK: Routledge.

Opie, I. & P. 1988. *The Singing Game*. Oxford: Oxford University Press.

Ornitz, E. M. 1989. 'Autism at the Interface Between Sensory and Information Processing'. In Dawson, G. (Ed). *Autism: Nature, Diagnosis and Treatment*. New York: Guilford.

Osborne, J. 2003. 'Art and the Child with Autism: Therapy or Education?'. In *Early Child Development and Care*. 173 (4). pp. 411–423.

Park, C. C. 1983. *The Siege*. London: Hutchinson & Co Ltd.

Piaget, J. 1962. *Play, Dreams and Imitation in Childhood*. New York: W. W. Norton.

—. 1982. *The Child's Conception of the World*. London: Granada Publishing Ltd.

Pietzner, Carlo (Ed). 1966. *Aspects of Curative Education*. Aberdeen: Aberdeen University Press.

Pietzner, Cornelius, (Ed). 1990. *A Candle on the Hill: Images of Camphill Life*. Edinburgh: Floris Books.

Poppelbaum, H. 1959. *Schicksalsrätsel*. Dornach.

Raffe, M. et al. 1974. *Eurythmy and the Impulse of Dance*. London: Rudolf Steiner Press.

Research Autism. July 27, 2012. 'Treatments and Therapies: Art, Art Therapy and Autism', from www.researchautism.net

Richardson, P. & J. 1994. 'Auditory integration training: how it helped our son'. *Communication*. 28 (1). pp. 9–12.

Richter, J. & Coates, S. (Eds). 2001. 'Meetings of Minds'. *Autism: The Search for Coherence*. p. 131.

Rimland, B. 1964. *Infantile Autism: The Syndrome and Its Implications for a Neural Therapy of Behaviour*. New York: Appleton Century Crofts.

—. 1996. *My 35 Years of Experience with Facilitated Communication*. San Diego: Autism Research Institute.

Roggenkamp, W. & Fischer, B. (Eds). 1974. *Healing Education Based on Anthroposophy's Image of Man*. Vereinigung der Heil und Erziehungs-Institute für Seelenpflege-bedürftige Kinder e.V. and Sozial-Therapeutische Werkgemeinschaft e.V.

Roth, I. 2010. *The Autism Spectrum in the 21st Century*. London: Jessica Kingsley Publishers.

Rubin, J. (Ed). 2001. *Approaches to Art Therapy*. UK: Brunner-Routledge.

Rutter, M. & Schopler E. (Eds). 1978. *Autism: a Reappraisal of Concepts and Treatment.* New York, London.

Rutter, M. & Howlin, P. 1989. *Treatment of Autistic Children.* John Oxford: Wiley & Sons.

Rutter, M. et al. 1994. 'Autism and known medical conditions: myth and substance'. *J. Child Psychology. 35* (2). pp. 311–22.

Sacks, O. 1986. *The Man who Mistook His Wife for a Hat.* London/Basingstoke: Picador, Macmillan.

—. 1994. 'An anthropologist on Mars'. *The New Yorker.* 27 December, 1993/3 January, 1994. pp. 106–25.

Sahlmann, L. 1969. *Autism or Aphasia. Developmental Medicine and Child Neurology. 2.* pp. 443–48.

Sanderson, N. & Fraley, G. 1994. 'Exchange of views'. *Communication. 28* (1). pp. 22–25.

Sandler, A. & colleagues. 9 December, 1999. 'Lack of benefit of a single dose of synthetic human secretin in the treatment of autism and pervasive developmental disorder'. *New England Journal of Medicine. 341* (24).

Schreibman, L. 1988. *Autism.* SAGE Publications.

Scotson, L. 1985. *Doran: Child of Courage.* London: Collins.

Seddon, R. 1988. *Rudolf Steiner, Essential Readings.* Crucible: The Aquarian Press.

Sellin, B. 1995. *In Dark Hours I Find My Way, Messages From An Autistic Child.* London: Victor Gollancz.

Shaddock, A. J., Spinks, A. T. & Esbensen, A. 2000. 'Improving Communication with People with an Intellectual Disability: the content validation of the Biala-II profile'. *International Journal of Disability, Development and Education. 47* (4). pp. 383–395.

Shattock, P. & Whiteley, P. 2000. *The Sunderland Protocol.* Durham conference paper, from osiris.sunderland.ac.uk/autism/durham2.htm

Sheridan, M. D. 1988. *From Birth to Five Years, Children's Developmental Progress.* NFER-Nelson.

SIGN (Scottish Intercollegiate Guidelines Network). 2007. Assessment, diagnosis and clinical interventions for children and young people with autism spectrum disorder. Scotland: NHS Education.

Simons, J. & Oishi, S. 1987. *The Hidden Child, the Linwood Method for Reaching the Autistic Child.* Rockeville: Woodbine House.

Siri, K. & Lyons, T. 2012. *Cutting-Edge Therapies for Autism*. New York: Skyhorse Publishing.

SLD (Support for Learning Division), School Directorate and Scottish Government. 2009. *The Autism Toolbox*. Edinburgh: Scottish Government.

Smith, T. 1995. *The Human Body*. London: Dorling Kindersley Limited.

Soesman, A. 1990. *The Twelve Senses*. Stroud: Hawthorn Press.

Stehli, A. 1991. *The Sound of a Miracle, a Child's Triumph over Autism*. New York: Doubleday.

Steiner, R. 1959. *The Inner Nature of Man, and the Life between Death and a new Birth*. London: Anthroposophic Publishing Company.

—. 1967. *A Lecture on Eurythmy*. London: Rudolf Steiner Press.

—. 1969a. *True and False Paths in Spiritual Investigation*. London: Rudolf Steiner Press.

—. 1969b. *Education as a Social Problem*. New York: Anthroposophic Press.

—. 1969c. *The Manifestations of Karma*. London: Rudolf Steiner Press.

—. 1970. *The Case for Anthroposophy*. London: Rudolf Steiner Press.

—. 1970a. *The Spiritual Guidance of Man*. New York: Anthroposophic Press.

—. 1970b. *At the Gates of Spiritual Science*. London: Rudolf Steiner Press.

—. 1972. *Curative Education*. London. Rudolf Steiner Press .(New edition published as Education for Special Needs in 1998).

—. 1973. *Theosophy, an Introduction to the Supersensible Knowledge of the World and the Destination of Man*. London: Rudolf Steiner Press.

—. 1975. *Life between Death and Rebirth*. New York: Anthroposophic Press.

—. 1975a. *The Education of the Child in the Light of Anthroposophy*. London: Rudolf Steiner Press.

—. 1976a. 'The work of the ego in childhood'. *Anthroposophic Quarterly*. 21 (4). pp. 86–92.

—. 1976b. *The Christ Impulse and the Development of Ego-Consciousness*. New York: Anthroposophic Press.

—. 1978. *The Effects of Spiritual Development*. London: Rudolf Steiner Press.

—. 1980. *Zur Sinneslehre*. Stuttgart.

—. 1981. *Man as a Being of Sense and Perception*. Vancouver: Steiner Book Centre.

—. 1982. *The Kingdom of Childhood*. London: Rudolf Steiner Press.

—. 1983. *Health and Illness. Volume 2*. New York: Anthroposophic Press.

—. 1986. *Soul Economy and Waldorf Education*.
London: Rudolf Steiner Press.

—. 1988. *The Child's Changing Consciousness and Waldorf Education*. London: Rudolf Steiner Press.

—. 1989. *Occult Science – an Outline*. London: Rudolf Steiner Press.

—. 1990a. *Learning to See into the Spiritual World*.
New York: Anthroposophic Press.

—. 1990b. *Study of Man*. London: Rudolf Steiner Press.

—. 1992. *The Philosophy of Spiritual Activity*.
London: Rudolf Steiner Press.

—. 1993. *Knowledge of the Higher Worlds, How is it Achieved?* London: Rudolf Steiner Press.

—. 1996. *The Foundations of Human Experience*.
New York: Anthroposophic Press.

—. 1997. (Lecture 9: August,1919) *Education as a Force for Social Change*. (GA 296) New York: Anthroposophic Press.

—. 1998. *Education for Special Needs*. London. Rudolf Steiner Press.

Steiner, R. & Wegman I. 1996. *Extending Practical Medicine*. London: Rudolf Steiner Press.

Stillman, B. 2006. *Autism and the God Connection*.
Naperville: Sourcebooks, Inc.

Stores, G. & Wiggs, L. June, 1998. 'Abnormal sleep patterns associated with Autism'. *Autism*. 2 (2).

Sulzer-Azaroff, B., Hoffman, A., Horton, C., Bondy, A. & Frost, L. 2009. 'The Picture Exchange Communication System (PECS) What Does the Data Say?'. *Focus on Autism and Other Developmental Disabilities*. 24 (2). pp. 89–103.

Sylva, K. & Lunt, I. 1982. *Child Development, a First Course*. Oxford: Basil Blackwell.

Taylor, B., Miller, E., Lingham, R., Simmons, A. & Stowe, J. 16 February, 2002. 'Measles, Mumps and Rubella Vaccination and Bowel Problems or Developmental Regression in Children with Autism: population study'. *British Medical Journal*. (324). pp. 393–396.

Tinbergen, N. & E.A. 1983. *Autistic Children, New Hope for a Cure*. London: George Allen & Unwin.

Trevarthen, C. 1987. 'Infancy, mind'. In Gregory, R. L., and Zangwill, O.L. (Eds). *Oxford Companion to the Mind*. Oxford: Oxford University Press.

Trevarthen, C., Aitken, K. J., Papoudi, D., and Robarts, J. Z. 1996. (2nd edition 1998). *Children with Autism, Diagnosis and Interventions to Meet their Needs*. London: Jessica Kingsley Publishers.

Tustin, F. 1992. *Autistic States in Children*. London & New York: Tavistock/Routledge.

Uhlenhoff, W. 2008. *The Children of the Curative Education Course*. Edinburgh: Floris Books

Verny, T. & Kelly, J. 1982. *The Secret Life of the Unborn Child*. London: Sphere Books.

Vieland (et al.). 2011. 'Novel method for combined linkage and genome-wide association analysis finds evidence of distinct genetic architecture for two subtypes of autism'. *Journal of Neurodevelopmental Disorders*. pp. 113–123.

Wachsmuth, G. 1937. *Reincarnation, as a Phenomenon of Metamorphosis*. Dornach: Philosophic-Anthroposophic Press.

Waring, R.H. May 2000. 'Suphation in Autism'. *Lecture at Autism Europe Congress*.

Weihs, T. J. 1975. 'The handicapped child – curative education'. In Davy, J. *Work arising from the life of Rudolf Steiner*.

—. 1984. *Children in Need of Special Care*. London: Souvenir Press.

Weirauch, Wolfgang (Ed). 2013. *Spiritual experiences of people with autism: Interviews with Hilke, Andreas, Erik and Martin Osika and Jos Meereboer*. Forest Row: Temple Lodge Publishing.

Whitehouse, A. February 5, 2012. 'DSM-V and the changing fortunes of autism and related disorders', from www.theconversation.com

Whiteley, P., Rodgers, J., Savery, D. & Shattock, P. March 1999. 'A Gluten-free Diet as an Intervention for Autism and associated Spectrum Disorders: preliminary findings'. *Autism*. 3 (1).

Williams, D. 1992. *Nobody Nowhere, the Extraordinary Autobiography of an Autistic*. New York: Times Books.

—. 1994. *Somebody Somewhere*. Doubleday.

—. 1998. *Autism An Inside-Out Approach*. London, England, and Bristol, USA: Jessica Kingsley.

Wiltshire, S. 1991. *Floating Cities*. London: Michael Joseph.

Wing, L. 1990. 'What is autism?' In Ellis, K. *Autism*.

—. 1993. *Autistic Continuum Disorders, an Aid to Diagnosis.* London: National Autistic Society.

—. 1996. *The Autistic Spectrum, a Guide for Parents and Professionals.* London: Constable.

Wood, D. 1988. *How Children Think and Learn.* Oxford: Basil Blackwell.

Woodward, R. S. 1985. *Aspects of the Waldorf* (Rudolf Steiner) School Curriculum as Offered in Schools for Normally Developing Children, and the Adaptation and Particular Contribution of this Curriculum for some Children with Special Educational Needs. University of Bristol Library (unpublished diploma dissertation).

Woodward, R. S. 1992. *Theory of Mind in the Light of Rudolf Steiner's Anthroposophy.* University of Bristol Library (unpublished M.Ed. thesis).

Zeedyk, S. 2006. 'From Intersubjectivity to Subjectivity: The Transformative Roles of Emotional Intimacy and Imitation'. *Infant and Child Development.* 15. pp. 321–344.

Zeylmans van Emmichoven, F. W. 1982. *The Anthroposophic Understanding of the Soul.* New York: Anthroposophic Press.

Ziviani, J. (Ed), Poulsen, A. & Cuskelly, M. 2013. *The Art and Science of Motivation: A Therapist's Guide to Working with Children.* London and Philadelphia: Jessica Kingsley.

Index

action plan 174f
adolescence 99
aggression 48, 107
aloofness 25, 27
American Psychiatric Association 31
anthroposophy / -ic 17, 52–96, 110,
   113, 150, 198–201, 204f, 227,
   242, 275–83
— interventions 112, 130
— medicine 54f, 117, 126
— model of autism 127, 155, 197
— therapists 123
— treatment 53
anti-fungal treatment 50
anxiety 167, 171
APGAR 128, 130
ARC model 165
art
— club 189–96
— therapy 123
Asperger, Hans 93, 216
Asperger syndrome 33, 92f
astral body see body, astral
Auditory integration training (AIT)
   102
autism
—, early infantile 25, 28f, 29, 92,
   234f
—, causes of 37–56, 239
—, primary 92, 200
—, secondary 92, 200
Autism Genome Project 39

Autistic Spectrum Disorder 33
Ayres, A. Jane 158, 267

Baird, Dr Gillian 30, 51
balancing activities 133
Baron-Cohen, Dr 42, 191
baths 270
—, foot 120, 270
—, hot 250
—, Pyrogenic 120
—, special 117
Bettelheim, Bruno 37, 81, 217, 242
bodily identity 167
body 228, 278
—, astral 65–67, 91, 112
—, etheric 65–67, 80, 91, 112
— geography 134, 137
— map 163
—, physical 65, 91, 112
— schemata 253, 264
Bogdashina, Olga 160f, 177, 182f,
   187
Bosch, G. 228, 234
brain
— development 41
— disorder 19
— function 41
— science 13, 15
— structure 40
breathing, regulating 167

Caldwell, Phoebe 159f, 165, 176f, 182
Campbell-McBride, Dr Natasha 44f
Camphill community school 17, 79, 83, 102, 109–11, 127–29, 179, 189, 243, 264
candida 45, 50
casein 45f, 48, 50f
characteristics 27
child development 59–75, 210, 231f, 236, 276
chirophonetics 286
Christ Event, the 63
Christian festivals 111
Clark, Robin P. 40
cognitive behavioural therapy (CBT) 103
colic 51
college meeting 126
communication 31, 34, 105f, 130, 141, 144, 146, 149, 180, 185, 194, 211, 253
compresses 54
consciousness, development of 229
constipation 19, 44, 48, 51
copy number variants (CNVs) 39
craft 261
— activities 225
— and work 122
Creak, Dr Mildred 29
curative education 109–55, 209, 218, 242–71
curriculum
—, school 120
—, Steiner-Waldorf 120f

Delacato 88, 158
diagnosis 28, 30, 32, 35, 216
—, differential 92, 200
—, early 209–26, 251
diarrhoea 19, 44, 48, 51, 54
diet 49, 51
—, exclusion 48, 50, 53

—, low sugar 50
—, low carbohydrate 50
digestion 19, 266
— problems 264
— process 43–56
Digestodoron tablets 54
drawing 117
DSM-5 19, 31–33, 88, 93
DSM-IV 33

early childhood 35. 227–42
— development 241f, 244, 282
echolalia 212f
education 101, 223f
—, Steiner-Waldorf 60, 165
EEG scan 43
ego 62, 64f, 67, 78, 91, 112, 147, 198, 229, 236, 276
ego-consciousness 214
ego-integration 42, 52, 55, 64, 67, 75, 77–79, 83, 90f, 94, 116, 118–21, 124f, 130, 141, 146, 151, 153, 200, 283
ego-organisation 42, 52, 54
Eisenberg, Leo 29, 37, 209, 239
endorphins 46
environmental factors 68
etheric
— body see body, etheric
— forces 79
eurythmy 115, 117, 119, 162, 166, 168, 249, 265f, 286
—, tone 269
executive function difficulties 171
exercises
—, lower sense 118
—, movement 265
—, resistance 118, 134, 264f
—, sensory 249
—, touch 267
eye contact 27, 73, 138f, 149, 211, 213f
eyes, black rings around the 51

facilitated communication (FC) 103
first year of life 12, 211f, 237
flatulence 48
food sensitivities 19
fourteen years of age 66

gastro-intestinal problems 48
genetics 38–40
genetic testing 43
gluten 45f, 48, 50f
Grandin, Temple 88f, 100, 157, 163, 177, 199
gravity 116, 264f
gross movement activities 132f, 135

Happé, Francesca 33
Hewett, Dr Dave 104, 159, 180–82
Hobson, Prof Peter R. 191
Hogenboom, Dr Marga 9, 13
hyperactivity 107
hypersensitivity 167
—, sensory 157
hyperventilation 133, 138f, 144, 148

ICD-10 31f, 83
Image of Man 59f, 74, 102, 113, 197f
imaginative play 28
imitation 28, 68, 78, 114, 127, 130, 212, 227, 229, 239, 268, 275f
incarnation 36, 66, 74f, 78, 90, 94, 125, 147, 154, 202, 239, 241, 282f
incidental teaching 104
individualisation 75, 94, 200, 202, 232f
intelligence 260
intensive behavioural intervention, early 103
interaction 34, 140, 149f
—, intensive 104, 162, 165, 179–88
—, peer 190
—, social 190
—, tactile 184

inter-human
— attitudes 112, 127, 130
— relationship 227, 235, 246
intervention, early 108

Jacobs, Paula 10, 179
joint attention 182, 185, 191f

Kanner, Leo 25, 28–30, 37, 83, 92, 130, 209, 227, 239
Kanner's syndrome 30, 92
karma 63–65, 83, 87, 90, 92, 202
Kaufman, Raun 26f, 105
Keller, Helen 280
König, Dr Karl 79–81, 84, 114, 227, 243

language processing disorder 171
large-headedness 83
Linwood method 102

massage 54, 125
—, rhythmical 125
mathematical-geometrical thinking 237
McAllen, Audrey 162
Mcbride, Dr Campbell 50
medical treatments 125
medication 107
melatonin 107
Merzenich, Dr Michael 158, 163
metabolic
— disorder 55
— processes 117
metabolic-limb system 61
metabolism 43–56, 266
milieu training 104
mood swings 107
moral issues 201
mother-child relationship 229, 231
MRI scan 43
Mukhopadhyay, Tito 158, 161f, 163
Müller-Wiedemann, Dr Hans 9, 13,

20, 79, 84–89, 115, 117, 207–71
music 119, 249, 270, 285f
— therapy *see* therapy, music

National Autistic Society 30
nerve-sense system 61
neurochemistry 42
neurodevelopmental
— disorder 38, 41
— movement 162
newborn 229, 239
NICE Guidelines 32, 43, 51, 55,
 102, 104
Nind, Prof Melanie 104, 180–82
normalisation 201f

obsessive
— actions 27, 139
— behaviour 141, 144f, 147 150,
 154
Olanzapine 107
Options method 105
Ornitz, E.M. 158

parents 108, 209–26, 247
Park, Elly 26, 85
Pedagogical Law 112
peptides 45f, 48, 51
personal pronouns 72, 82
phenol sulphur transferase 53
Piaget, Jean 68, 232, 241
picture exchange system (PECS)
 106f, 180, 184, 194f
pivotal response training (PRT) 106
play 73f, 79, 114f, 127, 130, 179,
 212, 268
—, therapeutic 179
— therapy *see* therapy, play
pre-birth existence 90, 92
prenatal 239, 241
proprioceptia 162, 164, 167
Provocation/Neutralization 100
pyrogenic 270

Reichelt, Dr Kalle 45
reincarnation 62, 202
repetitive
— behaviour 27, 31, 34, 115, 190,
 234
— speech 35
Research Autism 102
rhythmic 114
— activities 114, 127, 130
— system 123
rhythmical system 61, 135, 151
Rimland, Bernard 158
ring games 115
Risperidone 107
ritualised behaviour 35, 115, 264
rote-memory 28

sameness 27, 29, 238, 245, 254
Scherer, Stephen 40
schooling 223f
— special 102, 247, 248
Scottish Intercollegiate Guidelines
 Network (SIGN) 181
seven-year period 260
—, first 227, 236, 263
—, second 237, 259
—, third 260
second year of life 212
self-cognition 199
self-consciousness 72, 74, 79, 94f,
 231, 280
self-harm 107
self-isolation 29
Sellin, Birger 103
sense
— of balance 70, 116, 118, 162,
 236f, 263, 279
— of ego 71, 139, 281
— of hearing 71, 119
— of life 70, 116, 139, 163, 213,
 236f, 263, 266, 279
— of movement 70, 116f, 162, 236f,
 258f, 263, 265, 279

— of thought 71, 280
— of touch 70, 116, 118, 139, 162, 167, 235f, 263, 278
— of warmth 119, 150
— of word 71, 279
senses 88, 157–177
—, body *see* lower senses
—, higher 36, 69–71, 74, 78, 89, 130, 139, 199, 228f, 237, 258, 278
—, lower 69–71, 74, 78, 84f, 87, 89, 115, 130, 133f, 139, 144f, 161–163, 199, 214, 228, 233, 236f, 241, 249, 253, 263f, 278
—, middle 228, 236, 278
—, social 74
—, the twelve 89, 277f
sensory
— difficulties 157, 224
— input 35
— issues 34f
— organ 80f
— organisation 277
— overload 183
— perception 252
— profile 161, 183
— stimuli 28
sensory-perceptual development 115, 127, 130
Sensory Integration 158, 162, 174, 267
— therapy, *see* therapy, Sensory Integration
— problems 19, 171
serotonin 42
seventh year of life 66, 80, 233, 246
Shattock, Paul 45, 49
singing 115
sleeping problems 48
smiling 73, 138, 139, 229
social 34
— interaction 31
— life 94f
— pedagogy 89, 110f, 159, 180, 189

— skills 106
Social Stories™ 106
Son-Rise method 105
soul forces 60–62
spatial arrangements 228, 233, 235, 245
spectrum 30, 92, 200
speech 27, 99, 253, 257f
— disturbances 213
spiritual being 55, 62, 64, 74, 95, 155, 198, 202, 205, 280
Statens Serum Institut 43
Steiner, Rudolf 52f, 59f, 62–65, 67, 72f, 90, 112, 197, 199, 202–4, 209, 211, 214, 228, 237, 239, 241, 275–78
Steiner-Waldorf education *see* education, Steiner-Waldorf
stereotypical behaviour 218
Sterten, Mari 10, 157
Sunderland Protocol, the 49
Sunderland, University of 49
supplements 51
Surkamp, Johannes M. 10, 21
symmetry 235
symptoms, core 31

tactile stimulation 134
TEACCH Program 101f
testosterone 42
Theory of Mind 89, 181, 198
therapy
—, art 191, 195
—, coloured light 286
—, curative educational 263
—, eurythmy 124
—, holding 113
—, listening space 268f, 285
—, movement 184
—, music 105, 184
—, play 124, 249
—, riding 286
—, Sensory Integration 162

—, trumpet 285
—, warmth 250, 270
three years of life, first 25, 33, 36,
    68, 82, 216, 276, 278
third year of life 77, 212–15, 246,
    254
toddlers 12
Tóth, Réka 10, 189
touch activities 135
Trevarthen, Colwyn 17, 38
triad of impairments 31
turn-taking activities 135

Valtrex 100

video modelling 106f
visual schedules 106
— timetables 184
visual-spatial skills 28

Wegman, Dr Ita 52
Weihs, Dr Thomas 79, 82f
Whiteley, Paul 45, 49
Williams, Donna 48, 85, 88, 100,
    157, 177, 199, 205
Woodward, Bob 9, 13, 127, 157, 162
World Health Organisation 31

Zeedyk. 181, 185

Related books

Children with Special Needs
Rudolf Steiner's Approach

Michael Luxford

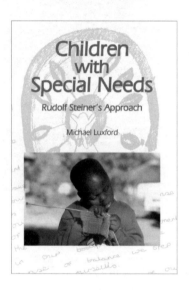

A concise and fully illustrated colour introduction to Rudolf Steiner's ideas on the development and education of children with special needs.

florisbooks.co.uk

Dyslexia
Learning Disorder or Creative Gift?

Cornelia Jantzen

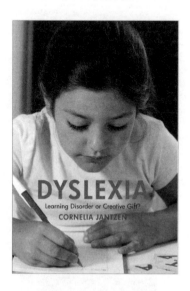

Explores the view that dyslexia is not a disability, but a special gift often coupled with a highly developed imagination and unique perception structure.

florisbooks.co.uk

The Children of the Curative Education Course

Wilhelm Uhlenhoff

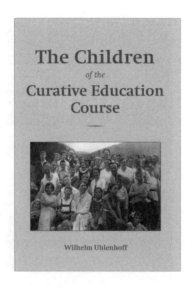

Seventeen detailed case studies of children with special needs and the effect of Rudolf Steiner's approach on their development.

florisbooks.co.uk

Discovering Camphill
New Perspectives, Research and Developments

Edited by Robin Jackson

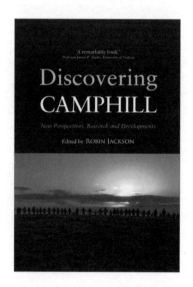

Brings together research from scholars and experts in a variety of disciplines to explore a broad range of issues which affect Camphill life.

florisbooks.co.uk

Books in the Karl König Archive

Vol 1: Karl König: My Task: Autobiography and Biographies

Vol 2: Karl König's Path into Anthroposophy : Reflections from his Diaries

Vol 3: Ita Wegman and Karl König: Letters and Documents

Vol 4: Child with Special Needs: Letters and Essays on Curative Education

Vol 5: Seeds for Social Renewal: The Camphill Village Conferences

Vol 6: Inner Journey Through the Year: Soul Images and the Calendar of the Soul

Vol 7: Calendar of the Soul: A Commentary

Vol 8: Becoming Human: A Social Task: The Threefold Social Order

Vol 9: Communities for Tomorrow

Vol 10: At the Threshold of the Modern Age: Biographies around the year 1861

Vol 11: Brothers and Sisters: The Order of Birth in the Family: An Expanded Edition

Vol 12: Kaspar Hauser and Karl König

Vol 13: Animals: An Imaginative Zoology

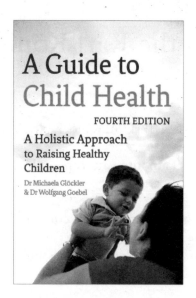

A Guide to Child Health

FOURTH EDITION

A Holistic Approach to Raising Healthy Children

Dr Michaela Glöckler & Dr Wolfgang Goebel

The Fourth edition of this comprehensive guide to children's physical, psychological and spiritual development. Combines medical advice with questions of development and education.

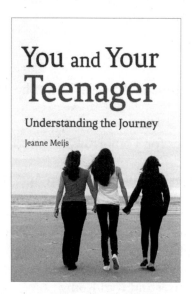

You and Your Teenager

Understanding the Journey

Jeanne Meijs

Seeing teenagehood as a journey along a path, ultimately to freedom, this book is both a considered overview of teenagehood and a practical, down-to-earth guide for parents facing particular challenges.